Pink Lemonade

Mastectomy Tips and Insights from a Breast Cancer Survivor

Martha,
Make your the day
Now and find joy
in every day!
Martha Lanier

Martha Lanier

Pink Lemonade
Mastectomy Tips and Insights from a Breast Cancer Survivor

Published by IGNITE Your Potential, Inc.
4990 Magnolia Creek Drive
Cumming, Georgia 30028

The information and tips in this book are presented in good faith and are for general information purposes only. All websites and phone numbers listed in this book are accurate at the time of printing, but may change or cease to exist in the future. The listing of website references and resources does not imply author endorsement of the site's entire contents. Groups and organizations are listed for informational purposes, and listing does not imply author endorsement of any of their activities.

All information is supplied with the understanding that the reader will perform their own due diligence and make their own determination as to its suitability for any purpose prior to any use of this information. The author, publisher and affiliated parties shall have neither liability nor responsibility to any person or entity with respect to any loss or damage caused or alleged to have been caused, directly or indirectly, by the information contained in this book. This publication is not intended to provide medical advice. Before making any decisions regarding health or wellbeing, consultation should be made with a member of the medical profession.

Back cover photograph: Shari Besher, Alpha Studios Inc
Front cover graphic and interior illustrations: Kristina Paquette
Design/layout: Rosamond Grupp

ISBN: 978-0-9819758-0-1

Printed in the United States of America

To my husband Jim, my children Liz Storch, Lauren Mills, Jim Lanier, Jr., their spouses, my seven incredible grandchildren and my sister, Linda Ward, who continue to provide endless support and encouragement.

To the many breast cancer survivors who have literally wrapped their arms around me and so graciously shared their experiences and positive attitudes.

To the women recently diagnosed with breast cancer who have unanswered questions and are just beginning their journey.

Table of Contents

Foreword

by J. Patrick Luke, M.D., F.A.C.S., General Surgery

The statistics are alarming. A woman has a one in eight chance of developing breast cancer in her lifetime. In 2008, 180,000 women were diagnosed with invasive breast cancer and another 60,000 to 70,000 were diagnosed with noninvasive breast cancer. There were 40,000 deaths reported in just this one year. It is these statistics that are the cause for anxiety every time a woman has a mammogram, a breast exam, or feels something unusual in her breast.

I have been a general surgeon in practice since 1987 and every week I have to tell patients, "Your biopsy shows a breast cancer." After providing this initial diagnosis, which is often overwhelming, we next discuss treatment options, further tests, prognosis, and recovery. Some forms of treatment encompass a host of medical factors as well as personal choices and perspectives giving the patient an opportunity to process and analyze her options.

Today there are many informative resources and support available that include family, friends, numerous books, and of course, the Internet. Unfortunately, much of the information comes across in a negative manner. Trying to sort through it all can be a daunting task in itself and can cause additional anxiety when trying to make the "right" decision. Patients must realize that there is not just one right decision. They must take into consideration medical and personal factors and make decisions that are best for them.

Martha Lanier gives a very candid and engaging account of her personal experiences from when she was first diagnosed with breast cancer through the details of her journey that followed. The information she provides is clinically informative, while at the same time positive and often humorous. Martha's content is presented in such a clear and positive manner that it makes the entire discussion and process much less intimidating. In addition, she provides insight and humor on many issues and nuances from a perspective that patients won't get from a discussion with their surgeon or oncologist.

Martha's book is a great resource for any woman who has been diagnosed with breast cancer or anyone who wants to offer support to a friend or family member who has been diagnosed. Despite all of the information available today, being diagnosed with breast cancer is still overwhelming for many people. Martha gives us an account that is real, refreshing, and positive.

Words from the Author

Two months shy of my 61st birthday, I was diagnosed with breast cancer. I felt totally unprepared as I entered this unfamiliar territory. Like most women, I never dreamed this would happen to me. But since it did, I sensed that it was my responsibility to learn as much as I could about breast cancer. That way, I could better understand what was ahead and be actively involved in the decisions that I had to make.

With each new experience, I kept saying, "Gee, I wish someone would've told me about this!" As a professional speaker, it is my habit to keep notes of my experiences so that I can share stories with my audiences and friends. It made sense for me to jot down my thoughts on sticky notes. The longer the process lasted, the more notes I accumulated. I had sticky notes on my computer monitor...on my bathroom mirror...on my refrigerator.

One day, while reading through my notes, it occurred to me, "Maybe I should write a book! If I write this down, other women won't be taken by surprise the way I was!"

Throughout the double mastectomy and reconstruction, I continued to write. While recuperating, I frequently sat on my screened porch organizing my notes. One afternoon I imagined a girlfriend sitting with me and sharing that she had just been diagnosed with breast cancer. That image gave me the courage to reveal more than is typical so that others may feel less isolated – particularly in the beginning. My idea for *Pink Lemonade* was born.

As you read these anecdotes and tips, my hope is that you will walk away informed, prepared, and entertained.

For your convenience, I've divided *Pink Lemonade* into three sections:

    I. My breast cancer story
    II. Tips I learned along the way
    III. My journal entries taken from my CaringBridge website

I must reiterate that this is *my* story. Not everyone would – or should – make the choices I made. It is based on information from my research from Internet websites, books, brochures, pamphlets, my surgical teams, and breast cancer survivors. All of the content is based on my memory, my interpretation of the events, and my own personal experiences.

The second section is filled with tips from my experiences and those of other breast cancer survivors. These tips are things that helped me cope, helped me feel better, and helped me survive. I share them with you from my heart.

This book is not intended to offer or recommend medical advice in any way. I am not suggesting you make the same decisions I did, but instead encourage you to make the choices you feel are best for you. Please consult with your doctors for their input on your specific circumstances. Every woman responds differently based on her individual diagnosis, emotions, healing, and recuperation. Although some breast cancer survivors' situations appear to be similar, they are each totally different.

My hope is that the following pages will stimulate your thought process to help you ask more questions and understand the value that comes with knowledge. Knowledge comes from research, the expertise of your medical teams, and experience.

Martha

Section I

Prologue

CHAPTER 1

My Story

Prior to the spring of 2008 when I was diagnosed with breast cancer, I could count on one hand the number of women (or men) I personally knew who had also been diagnosed. When I was growing up, Mrs. Malone lived just two houses down from us on the same side of our street. At the time, she had three adorable little girls whom I loved to baby-sit. They were the type of family that was close and always doing something fun. After I married and moved out of town, she was diagnosed with breast cancer. I remember my mom telling me that she had undergone a mastectomy (without reconstruction). I couldn't wait to come back into town so I could sit and visit with her. When I saw her, she was propped up in bed and surrounded with fluffy white pillows. Although she still had the same cheerful smile, I remember being surprised at how sick she was.

That was when I made the decision that if I were ever diagnosed with cancer, I would refuse treatment and just let nature take its course. Isn't it funny how we always think we know exactly what we would do if we were in a particular situation? That is, until we get there. Then in a split-second we change our minds and do the exact opposite.

Some 40 years later, when I was diagnosed with cancer, I totally disregarded my earlier decision. At that point all I could think about was living.

Life Is Good

It was still dark outside when my alarm buzzed. No hitting the snooze! I was wide-awake. That day I was on top of the world! I was to be interviewed in a guest spot on Atlanta's 11Alive News on WXIA (NBC). It was April 1, 2008, and I had been asked to provide tips to help all of metro Atlanta clean their clutter and get organized for spring. I was sure Oprah would be calling me next!

To celebrate my (imagined) fame, later in the day my daughter, Liz and her three boys would be arriving from Spartanburg, South Carolina. Okay, they really didn't know I was going to be famous; they were just coming for spring break. Topping off the day, I was speaking that evening to a networking group on how to stay focused and positive. It was bound to be a long day, but I was excited. I was doing work that I loved and spending time with my family. It just doesn't get any better than that. I thought, "Life is good ... really good!"

The TV interview went well, but (perhaps not surprisingly) Oprah didn't call. Even though I was pressed for time, I stopped by T.J. Maxx on my way home, adding an extra errand into an already full day. As I pulled my car into a parking space, my cell phone rang. It was a call from my internist.

"I would like for you to have another chest x-ray. The one taken last week during your annual physical is not totally clear. I've seen this happen before and I really don't think there is anything to worry about, but it's better to be sure."

I scheduled the appointment for the Friday after my daughter and the boys left. I saw no reason to interrupt our fun for something so routine.

The day continued as planned; little did I realize at the time that it was going to be a day I would long remember.

A Day of Discovery

Just before going to bed that same night, while rubbing lotion across my chest, I felt a slight, soft bulge above my right breast. At first, I thought it was just a muscle. I felt my left breast to see if perhaps I was developing asymmetrically ... before remembering that I was 50 years past puberty. There was no sign of a similar bulge on the left side. I was not overly concerned and made a mental note (which I hoped I would remember) to tell my doctor about it on Friday while having my chest x-ray repeated. It was no big deal.

Fortunately, my second chest x-ray was negative, but my doctor was quite concerned about the lump I had found and the fact that it wasn't detected during my previous visit. During that visit, my breast exam was performed with me lying down. The lump could only be felt when I was sitting or standing. Although my doctor believed it was a small mass consisting of just fatty tissue, she ordered a mammogram and ultrasound. I am forever thankful she chose to take an aggressive approach. Without her actions, it could have been years before my cancer was found.

Driving to my appointment, I thought back on how I used to dread mammograms. It wasn't just the discomfort, but the panic attacks. My breast would be reconfigured to resemble a disposable paper plate held securely in place between two ice-cold sledgehammers. What did they think, I might escape and run bare-breasted through the halls? Once locked into place, panic would set in as I envisioned the fire alarm piercing the silence of the hospital just after the technician left the room to "take the picture" so she could avoid the radiation. There I would be – abandoned, flattened into place, hugging a frigid piece of metal. With this horrifying thought, I would beg the technician to talk to me continuously the entire time she was out of sight so I would know she had not deserted me. Thank goodness today's machines have an automatic release, and with digital mammography, the technicians never leave the room.

About ten years ago, I changed to a new medical facility where the mammogram technician went to great lengths to minimize the discomfort and still get a clear image. Too bad she can't be cloned. Since then, I almost—but not totally—don't mind the ordeal and actually look forward to seeing her. Besides, she is like an old friend I only get to see once a year.

That day we exchanged friendly small talk. I showed her the fatty tissue in question. Three different times she used all her strength to pull and stretch my skin so she could capture an image of my mysterious little fatty tissue, but because it was situated so high on my chest wall, it was just not possible.

Disappointed that she wasn't able to get an image of it, she walked me across the hall to the ultrasound room. My new tech performed the ultrasound and soon left the room to discuss the results with the radiologist. She returned with a smile, telling me I was free to leave. Her parting words were, "If there are any significant findings, your doctor will get in touch with you." Although I was not told at the time, the ultrasound did reveal something suspicious inside "my little fatty tissue."

Suspicions

Completely unconcerned, I flew to Seattle the following day to give the opening keynote at a women's conference. The audience was wonderful and the program a success. Pleased with the results of my presentation, I took a cab to the airport to fly back to Atlanta. It had been another great day.

At airport security, I put my jacket, purse, shoes, and cell phone in a bin on the security conveyor belt. Just as my possessions were disappearing into the dark cavern of the x-ray machine, my cell phone rang. With a quick glance, I saw my internist's name pop up on the caller ID and immediately felt a weird sensation in the pit of my stomach. I grabbed my phone and yelled, "I'm going through airport security; call me right back!"

Fortunately, I quickly made it through security and found an unoccupied gate. After waiting for what seemed an eternity, my phone finally rang again. I heard her say, "The results of your ultrasound revealed a questionable area that needs to be checked. I want you to see a breast surgeon as soon as possible. If you don't know of one, I can recommend one." I quickly explained I would only be home for the night and would be flying back out early the next morning for a weekend conference. I wouldn't be home until Monday night. I promised to make an appointment as soon as I got back.

For the first time, I felt a little concern ... a slight uncertainty. So far, I had not shared any of my office visits, repeat x-ray, mammograms, or ultrasound with anyone, including my husband, Jim. He had so many things on his mind; I just didn't see a need for him or anyone else to worry unnecessarily. Also, I didn't want to risk having anyone look at me and wonder if I had cancer, or worse yet, ask me every day if the fatty tissue had grown, how I was doing, or if I was concerned or scared. It was my little secret and I liked knowing something no one else knew. Besides, there still was no reason to think it was all that serious.

Unexpected News

The next thing on my to-do list, having nothing to do with the "breast" situation, was to see my gynecologist for my annual exam. My appointment just happened to be on the same morning as my first appointment with the breast surgeon. Of course, I told my gynecologist about my new lump. She examined it and said, "That's probably just some fatty tissue. Nothing I would worry about."

To add even more confusion to my medical history, she did show concern about some minor post-menopausal spotting I was having. To my surprise, she insisted I have a D&C as soon as possible. I left her office feeling less concerned about my little fatty tissue and more concerned about having the D&C.

I had just enough time for a quick lunch before my appointment with the breast surgeon. As soon as I entered his office, his staff treated me more like a friend than a patient. It was just what I needed at the time. When the doctor walked into the examining room, I liked him immediately. He had a gentle voice, a warm smile, and a genuine persona. After he examined my little fatty tissue, he suggested I have a core needle biopsy, which is generally the first procedure performed for tissue diagnosis. It is less invasive and often avoids a surgical procedure, plus it would allow him to know exactly what he was dealing with before considering surgery.

Instead, I asked if he could surgically remove it. By this time, I was tired of feeling the lump on a daily (if not hourly) basis. My thinking was that I just didn't want it anymore, cancer or no cancer. His impression was that clinically, my lump did not appear worrisome. Based on this fact and my concern, he agreed to an excisional biopsy (surgically removing the lump). For once I felt empowered and in control.

So, I found myself scheduled for an excisional biopsy on Monday, April 28 and a D&C on the following Monday, May 5th . If both ended up requiring additional surgery, I was wondering, which would come first, a mastectomy or a hysterectomy? It was sort of like the chicken and the egg.

'Fessing Up

Once I realized my situation had gone from routine to questionable, I was having second thoughts about not having shared all of the details – really *any* of the details -- with Jim, going all the way back to my annual exam.

As you might have guessed by now, in many ways I am a rather private person and I also like being in control. Because anesthesia was required for each procedure, I realized someone would have to drive me to and from the hospital. So it was time to either tell Jim … or explain why a taxi was picking me up and returning me home a little groggy on two consecutive Mondays. That didn't sound like something a husband would easily ignore, and definitely not Jim.

For the next few days, I focused on my speaking engagements, completing my commitments one by one. On the way home from the last scheduled speech, I puzzled over what I was going to say to Jim. How could I explain the scary news and such short notice all at the same time?

"Are you available to drive me to the hospital next Monday so I can have a little fatty tissue removed from my breast? And by the way, the following week, I'll need you again because I'm having a D&C. How's this work with your schedule?"

It's just not that easy writing those kinds of speeches.

I rehearsed over and over again all the way home, even changing the inflection in my voice to see if it would soften the message. When I walked in the house, I found Jim in his favorite glider, relaxing on our screened porch. I joined him and we started talking about really important things like the weather, dinner and our grandchildren, while I tried to find the perfect time to begin.

Finally, in a rather casual voice, I said, "By the way, I found a lump in my right breast and have decided to just go ahead and have it removed. Both my internist and surgeon think it is probably just a little fatty tissue, but they want to check it out to make sure. I'm really not worried about it myself."

It was obvious Jim was still processing what he had just heard when I started to speak again. By then my voice indicated I might be a little tense and nervous. In the next breath, I said, "Oh yeah, I've also been to see my gynecologist …"

Before I could say more, he leaned toward me and yelled, "Don't tell me you're pregnant!"

While staring intensely at each other, we both burst out laughing at the ridiculous thought of two 60-year-olds becoming parents all over again! After all, we already had three children and seven grandchildren. With a smile on my face and a new sense of calmness, I was able to share with him the details of the previous three weeks. His humor was a tremendous help in easing what was once a tense moment.

I assured Jim that I was not worried … and I really wasn't. Because I didn't panic, he didn't panic. I honestly believe that emotions are contagious. I was grateful that Jim took the cue from me. I'm sure he was concerned, but at least for the next two weeks our lives went on as usual.

Excisional Biopsy

Although we arrived at the hospital on time for my excisional biopsy, my surgery was delayed for several hours due to a prior procedure taking longer than anticipated. When I woke up, Jim told me that the surgeon had removed the small mass and still believed it was nothing more than "a little fatty tissue." It would be sent to pathology for further testing, and I could call the surgeon's office on Thursday to learn the results.

Jim and I headed for home and I slept like a baby through the night. For the next several days I was sore, but it was nothing I couldn't handle. I was soon back to my usual activities and energy level.

Before the biopsy, I had been calm and basically unconcerned. I had never seriously thought I might have cancer. My father was a heavy smoker and had died from lung cancer; I had no other family history of cancer and I'd had negative mammograms for the past fifteen years.

As I was lying in bed planning my day the morning after the biopsy, reality hit. I thought to myself, "You'd better quit putzing around, get your act together, and learn as much as you can, just in case the pathology report reveals you *do* have breast cancer."

I spent literally all day Tuesday and Wednesday glued to the Internet, reading anything and everything I could about breast cancer from diagnosis to treatments such as lumpectomies and mastectomies.

The Long Wait

Thursday turned out to be an extremely long day. I waited and waited -- until 9:10 a.m. to call my surgeon's office. I thought he would have a good ten minutes to review my report and talk to me before he started seeing patients. His assistant answered and said he had not arrived, but she expected him any minute and would have him return my call. By 11:00 I still hadn't heard from him and assumed he was busy seeing patients, but I tried calling again. This time, his assistant told me he was with a patient and would definitely return my call. When I asked if she knew if he had received my pathology report, she confirmed it was on his desk and that he would call me as soon as he could.

By then my mind had started playing games with me. The longer I waited, the more certain I became that the news was not going to be good. Besides, if the report had been negative, then a quick phone call from his assistant would have solved it. Explaining I had breast cancer would obviously take much longer. He would probably wait until he finished seeing his patients.

Just after 4:00, my breast surgeon finally called. For the first time in my life, I kept my mouth shut and I listened patiently.

"Martha, the pathology report reveals that a small 0.7 centimeter cancer was found inside the fatty tissue that was removed. The good news is that it was found early and is very small. Because of this, you will have several options."

Cancer. You never know how you're going to react when you hear that word spoken directly to you. For many women it brings tears, a range of emotions, doubts, fear, panic. If you do feel any of these, it's okay. Go ahead and cry or scream. You will have your own way of coping. It's okay. You may want to call everyone you know or keep it to yourself. Either way, it's okay.

Some women I meet say they didn't feel these emotions and remained calm while their relatives and friends seemed to fall apart. It doesn't mean that they are unemotional, it just happens to be the way they chose to deal with being diagnosed with cancer.

For me, I have always faced fear or challenges by turning my focus in a totally different direction such as research and looking for solutions. This is how I choose to keep my mind from wondering in a negative direction. In the Tips section, I mention a meltdown I had shortly after being diagnosed.

If you hear the word cancer, whatever your response, whatever you do, however you feel…*any* emotion is okay. This is a woman's prerogative.

After telling me the diagnosis, my doctor explained that he was leaving for a mountain climbing adventure in Alaska in two days. (I liked him even more when I realized we both enjoyed exciting adventures). Rather than delay this discussion for more than ten days, he offered to meet with Jim and me at 8:00 the next morning. I will always appreciate his concern and thoughtfulness in meeting with me right away to answer my immediate questions.

After we hung up, I thought how much I liked the manner in which he told me, and that he didn't make me wait until the following morning in his office. That gave me some personal time alone to process my new identity—breast cancer survivor.

Back to Reality

Several minutes later, I looked at my watch and realized that if I hurried, I could still make my hair appointment. Like any normal woman, I certainly didn't want to miss it and have to reschedule.

While quickly driving the back roads to my hairdresser, I called Jim first, then our three children, and then my sister to tell them the news, "I have breast cancer. Because it is small and was found early, I have options." It was strange, but I wasn't upset and had a strong feeling I was going to be okay.

At the hair salon, I quietly worked in my Sudoku book while my mind was racing, trying to remember everything I had so diligently researched. I acted like nothing was different. After all, I was the same person I had always been. Having cancer wouldn't change that.

I was still not ready to tell anyone other than my immediate family. I wanted to process my new challenge and work on developing my plan before sharing it with the world. I remember being surprised at my calmness. In fact, I actually felt an inner peace. I realized I was experiencing the miracle of my faith. I was not afraid, nervous, or uptight. I felt confident and as prepared as any woman could be. My plan began to unfold. Although it was a preliminary plan, it was all mine. Again, I felt I was in total control.

Diagnosis

Early Friday morning, May 2, my surgeon met with Jim and me for almost an hour. Because I am a visual person, I appreciated that he gave me the pathology report to read for myself. Focusing on each word, I read, "3.5 by 2.0 by 1.7 centimeter fibrofatty breast tissue" (here we go again with the fatty tissue) "contains a 0.7 centimeter lesion. Final Pathologic Diagnosis: INFILTRATING WELL DIFFERENTIATED DUCTAL CARCINOMA (0.7 CM)." If you are not into metrics, the mass was roughly the size of half a large squished marshmallow and the lesion was less than half the size of a Tic-Tac breath mint.

He told me that because my cancer was small and had been detected early, I could have additional tissue removed from the biopsy site, leaving a clear margin around where the cancer had been, and then follow with six weeks of radiation. This is a choice made by many women with the same diagnosis. I stopped him there and told him about my research and the first part of my plan.

"I have made the decision to treat it aggressively and have a bilateral mastectomy." My reasoning was that at age 60 I didn't have a problem having both of my breasts removed. My own theory was that perhaps this might decrease the chances of developing cancer in my other breast years from now.

He suggested I talk with other breast cancer survivors whose treatments included lumpectomies and radiation, single mastectomies, bilateral mastectomies, reconstruction using artificial implants, and reconstruction with implants formed from their own tissues. I had no idea I would have so many choices. He also gave me the names of several plastic surgeons (which he does with all his breast cancer patients), and suggested I see more than one unless I was confident with the first one I saw. He explained he would be working closely with whomever I chose because he advises having the mastectomy and reconstruction performed at the same time to avoid a second surgery later on. He told me to ask what form of reconstruction each of them would suggest was suitable specifically for me. I left his office that morning with the additional information necessary to proceed with my plan.

The following week was already filled with medical visits. Monday was the D&C. On Wednesday, the biopsy stitches were being removed and I had an appointment with my first potential plastic surgeon. On Friday, I would have an MRI to rule out the possibility of cancer being found in my other breast.

On Monday, the D&C revealed nothing significant, which meant no hysterectomy. Whew! I could forget about my bottom half and concentrate on my top half. Having the stitches removed from the biopsy incision was a piece of cake, although I admit I was so nervous it was going to hurt. It didn't hurt at all. My consultation with the first plastic surgeon left me apprehensive and unsure about having a mastectomy and reconstruction. I thought, maybe I should reconsider the lumpectomy and radiation.

Search for a Plastic Surgeon

The following Monday I had a consultation with a second plastic surgeon. The majority of breast cancer survivors I talked to told me I should definitely meet with him before making my decision.

I didn't care if my surgeon was a male or a female. What did matter was having someone who was sensitive and personable. I wanted someone who would not hesitate to answer my questions regardless of how insignificant they might seem. I wanted someone who was professional, yet had a good sense of humor. I knew that if I did decide to have the mastectomy, I wanted the surgeon to use my own tissues for the implant by having an abdominal TRAM. Therefore, my number-one priority was finding a surgeon who had the most experience and a high rate of success with this procedure.

The TRAM (transverse rectus abdominal muscle) was developed by Dr. C.R. Hartrampf, who had been the second plastic surgeon's senior partner before he retired. The TRAM procedure is similar to having a tummy tuck. The tissue that is removed from the abdomen is used to form the breast implants. The success of this procedure depends on intricate microscopic surgery to reconnect the blood vessels and keep the tissues alive.

The first time I met with this particular plastic surgeon, he made me feel like I was his one and only patient. He spent so much time explaining what I could expect in great detail, from the initial surgery through my recovery, as well as long-term results. He never hesitated to answer all of my questions, even going so far as to draw pictures all over the paper on the examining table. Because of his years of experience performing the TRAM and the fact that he learned from the surgeon who developed the procedure, I had confidence in him and totally trusted his ability. He smiled and assured me I would be pleased with the results. It was so easy to see how passionate he was about helping women feel good about themselves throughout the entire process.

Although he was not one of the surgeons listed with my insurance company, I knew he was definitely the surgeon I wanted for this procedure. Eight years earlier, I had purchased a supplemental cancer policy with Aflac. It turned out to be one of the best decisions I could have made. Having this additional insurance coverage made it financially possible to use a surgeon who was not with our health insurance plan. I didn't have to be concerned with the out-of-pocket expense and the additional funds I received gave me a boost.

There was no doubt in my mind that this plastic surgeon would do an incredible job reconstructing my new breasts. Everyone in his office was also wonderful. Again, I felt like I was receiving special treatment. His scrub nurse anticipated many of my questions and was generous in sharing ideas based on previous patients' experiences. She was definitely an added bonus to the surgical team, but then again, each of his nurses and administrative staff was great.

Once I made my final decision to have a bilateral mastectomy with reconstruction using implants from my abdomen, I realized the lemons I had been given were turning into lemonade! And in honor of all breast cancer survivors, I decided my lemonade from there on out would always be pink!

Renewed Confidence

Finally, I was confident I had two incredible surgical teams in place. My bilateral mastectomy and reconstruction were scheduled for 7:00 a.m. on Tuesday, June 3, 2008.

My next step was to put the second phase of my plan into place. I told all of my friends either by phone or email that I had breast cancer and that I needed their help. I set up a website on CaringBridge (see section three) and gave everyone the link. For me it was easier telling them this way because I didn't have to repeat the details of the experience to each one of them. As a speaker, nothing I ever say is brief, and there simply were not enough hours in the day or week for me to explain everything to everyone. Also, I didn't want to create an uncomfortable situation for friends if I told them face-to-face, especially when I didn't know what their responses would be. Personally, I wasn't sure I was prepared to handle the expressions on their faces, which could have revealed shock, sadness, and sorrow. This was just my way of dealing with it.

I asked my friends for three things:

- Prayers for strength to face whatever came my way. I also asked for prayers for my family and for the skills and abilities of my surgical teams.
- Humor to make me laugh. I planned on using laughter throughout my healing process.
- Help in eliminating stress in my life. In other words, "Don't ask me to serve on, much less chair, a committee of any sort anytime soon."

I made a commitment that I would no longer allow myself to become stressed over anything! I soon became known as "Mellow Martha." I also focused on maintaining a positive attitude. I avoided anyone who happened to be having a bad day or who was naturally negative.

My personal goal was to be in the best physical condition I could be in prior to surgery. Early on, I started walking every morning in our neighborhood. By the day before my surgery, I was walking a brisk three miles in 50 minutes. I know some people may not think that was so great, but for a non-athlete, I think it was extraordinary, especially for someone who doesn't like to sweat!

On the night prior to surgery, I was confident that I was as prepared as anyone could be—mentally, physically, and spiritually. I was ready to get the show on the road so I could soon sit back and enjoy a nice cool drink of pink lemonade!

Section II

Tips

CHAPTER 2

Diagnosis

Many women depend on the strength of their family and close friends when facing potentially shocking news, especially when it is about their health. I can't explain why my attitude is so different, but I prefer to process in private. The only explanation I have is that for most of my life, it was my mother's nature to make decisions for me. I loved her dearly, but I learned to keep my thoughts and feelings to myself rather than risking the opposition that could come with voicing them. Internalizing my thoughts is what gives me the feeling of being in control— of my emotions, my thoughts, and my reactions.

My desire to keep the news to myself deepened when I thought about how I would maintain a positive attitude as I faced concerned responses from my family and friends. Ever since I was a child, I have been accused of looking at life through rose-colored glasses. I am a dreamer and think of the "what if's" as adventures. My "glass" isn't merely half-full, it's overflowing -- that's how I choose to embrace life. This is how I maintain a positive attitude, which gives me energy. Negative attitudes—whether mine or someone else's—totally zap my energy and leave me feeling down and exhausted.

I try to avoid anything that may deplete my energy, even if it is the concerns of those who love me.

One of the things that depletes the energy of so many who experience breast cancer is a feeling that they don't know what to do, where to go, or how to feel when certain things happen. When I *found out, I looked for a "How to Have a Mastectomy" book with step-by-step guidelines, but I never could find one. So for the rest of the book, I will be offering tips so that you will not feel alone, unsure, or confused about what to do. These tips are based on my own experiences and the experiences of others. You may or may not find your experiences to be the same as mine. I offer these tips in the hope that they will help you feel informed and empowered.*

Personal Time

TIP: Give yourself time to process what you have learned and the feelings you are experiencing. For some women, it may be talking and sharing your thoughts with friends and family. For others, it may be spending some personal time alone to reflect and think. What is most important is that you give yourself the time to do what works best for you.

Shortly after receiving the news that I had breast cancer, I was standing in a long checkout line where the majority of shoppers were women. As I looked at each of those women, I wondered how many of them might also be breast cancer survivors.

Over and over again I silently repeated in my mind, "I have breast cancer." I slowly graduated to saying it out loud—in the car, in the shower and when I was alone at home. Practicing was a tremendous help and soon the words flowed smoothly and were much easier to say.

I found comfort during my quiet times, when I prayed for strength and thought about how many different ways I could benefit from my experience. I learned more about who I really am and what I believe than most people learn in their entire lifetime. And I knew I was going to be just fine.

Meltdowns

---------------------------- 〜✿〜 -----------------------------

TIP: **Regardless of how strong you are or how pre-pared you are, sometimes a single word or look can trig-ger a meltdown when you least expect it. It's okay. No one can be strong every single minute of every day.**

Right from the beginning, I was able to maintain focus and stay in control. Then the unthinkable happened.

I was talking on the phone with a customer service representative from the pharmacy of our health insurance company. I had just received a letter stating that my refill for Boniva had been denied. Boniva is the once-a-month pill for osteoporosis. When I asked why I was not able to get a refill, especially since I had been taking it for over a year, I was told in a rather firm voice, "*You* have been *declined.*"

I have always been well known for being calm and easygoing; rarely do I ever raise my voice or lose my cool. Without warning, the flood-gates opened and I barely stopped short of sobbing uncontrollably. "I can handle feeling old and post menopausal. I can even handle being told I have breast cancer. But I can't handle being told I've been *de-clined* a prescription refill for medication that will help me be like Sally Field." Since my only audible sounds were no longer recognizable, I hung up. Never in my life have I ever been so thoughtless as to hang up on someone.

After several minutes my phone rang. It was the customer service rep calling back. She told me that her mother was a breast cancer survi-vor, and she wished me well. She explained that the denial had nothing to do with me personally, but that my insurance company no longer ap-proved Boniva for anyone. I really appreciated the fact that she took the time to call me back, especially after being on the receiving end of my meltdown.

Telling Family and Close Friends

──────────────── こ未ら ────────────────

TIP: **Some women immediately need the support of family and friends. Others need personal time to process what is happening. Trust your instincts.**

Initially, I had an easier time saying "cancer" than I did "breast." Being 60, I grew up in a time when you never said the word breast in public, much less in mixed company ... or even at home! My mother simply would not allow it. We would just point to what concerned us. In fact, it wasn't until long after my children were born that I was able to use the correct names for all body parts, and then it would still embarrass me.

Telling friends either by phone or by email seemed better than pointing to my right breast and saying, "I have cancer ... here." This may have been the chicken's way out, but it was the best way for me to share the news. I didn't know how they were going to respond, and I didn't want to see their facial expressions.

I only told three people face-to-face, because they all happened to be standing together. I was thinking there would be safety in numbers, not realizing until too late that *they* had the numbers – I was on my own. I was nervous and tried to think of an easy way to break the news. At a pause in the conversation, I casually said, "By the way, I've been diagnosed with breast cancer." There was immediate silence as all three of them stared at me with looks of shock and disbelief. It was obvious they had no idea what to say. That's when I realized that sharing my news might dredge up unexpected, unpleasant memories of a relative's or close friend's experience with cancer.

I decided that from that day forward, I would only let people know by phone or email. That would cut down on the potential discomfort for them and for me.

It's surprising, but I had no problem telling total strangers. In fact, I told everyone who came within talking distance. I wore a pink ribbon pin and bracelet, which frequently generated conversations while I was waiting in line or shopping. Total strangers would see my pink ribbon and share a smile or a gentle hug and offer their support; most of the time they identified themselves as breast cancer survivors and shared great tips or offered words of encouragement. To me this was extremely comforting.

Support System

━━━━━━━━━ ❧❦❧ ━━━━━━━━━

TIP: Take someone with you to your key appointments. Choose someone you respect and who genuinely cares about you. These are times when you can definitely use an extra pair of ears to help you remember new and important information.

My mind was constantly processing everything I was being told. I wanted to make sure I remembered even the smallest details.

My husband Jim went with me whenever I asked him. He is my best friend and biggest supporter. We have been friends since we met in the fifth grade, and after almost 40 years of marriage, we know each other well. He is my number one supporter.

After my surgeon discussed the pathology report in detail and I said I wanted to have a bilateral mastectomy, Jim looked me right in the eye and without hesitation said, "I support you 100% in whatever treatment you want to have."

I love that he never questioned my decision nor tried to talk me out of having a bilateral mastectomy. This is what true friends will do for each other, especially when they know you have done your homework and you have considered all of your options.

Set the Tone

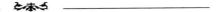

> TIP: **Your attitude sets the tone. I believe that people will mirror the actions they see. It is harder for friends to be overly upset if you maintain a positive and upbeat attitude and set the example of how you wish to be treated. If a conversation loses positive energy, speak up and tell friends you are counting on them for their positive support.**

I have always heard, "Attitudes are contagious," and in my life, it's absolutely true! When friends and family realized I was not down or uptight, they seemed to relax.

In the past when someone would share surprising news with me, I would watch them for clues to how I should react or what I should say.

When I found myself on the flip side, I focused on staying positive and not stressed. I tried to let others know through my actions that I was okay and staying positive.

Be Your Own Advocate

> TIP: **Use your knowledge, your common sense, your gut feelings, your intuition, and any means you have to stay true to yourself in the decisions you will be making. Don't let anyone talk you out of or into doing anything you don't feel is right for you.**

I grew up during a time when as a woman I was taught to accept what I was told, especially by an authority figure. Today I know to ask more questions and do my own research before agreeing to do what someone else suggests I do.

Know your body and listen to your intuition. Use your research. It is said that knowledge is power, but I say it is what you *do* with your knowledge that is empowering.

Talk to other breast cancer survivors and ask them questions about their experiences, the size and type of their cancer, and their treatment. Ask your hospital if they offer a breast cancer support group. Often they have breast cancer survivors on standby to answer your questions.

Whether you have just found a lump, have discovered something suspicious, or know you may be facing surgery, you can always get a second or even third opinion. What is most important is that you have total confidence in your doctors and your decision.

I learned never to stop learning and to *ask, ask, ask!*

Medical Records and Pathology Reports

TIP: **You have a right to all of your medical records. Ask for copies of reports from your office visits and physical exams, as well as all lab, x-ray, pathology, operative, and other medical records. They belong to you.**

I have a copy of every single report related to my diagnosis and treatment, from the lab reports from my initial physical to the operative reports from my last surgery. I wanted to know all of the details, whether I could interpret every report or not. When a question about a procedure occurred to me, I was able to locate and read the report immediately.

In the beginning, I had a single hardcover file folder for my records, and I thought I was so organized! Before long, I added a second folder, and within weeks, I switched to an accordion file folder with multiple pockets. I noticed a number of other women would bring accordion files with them to their appointments, and realized I wasn't alone in my record keeping.

I took this file with me to all of my doctors' appointments, even though I didn't need to do so. Maybe it gave me confidence to know I could look something up on my own. It also provided a safe place for me to keep my list of questions and write down answers.

MRI

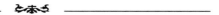

TIP: **If you are going to have an MRI, ask at the time of scheduling if it will be done in an open or closed cylinder. If you think you may not be able to relax in a closed cylinder due to claustrophobia, ask your doctor for medication that will help you relax and tolerate the procedure. If you do take something to help you relax, you will likely need to have someone drive you to and from the procedure.**

Although I am not afraid to jump out of a plane when skydiving, I have always been claustrophobic. A few years ago, I faced my first MRI with my trademark positive attitude, and reassured myself it wasn't going to be a bad experience. To show the technician how calm I was about the MRI, I told her I planned on taking a nap while I was in there. Because she didn't want to disturb me, she never spoke, but instead had soft music playing through my earphones. After several minutes, I opened my eyes for one quick peek and wished I hadn't. I felt like my eyelashes were inches from touching the top. When I tried to relax, my elbows would slowly slide outward and touch the sides. It was just too close for me. I felt like I had been buried alive.

By the time the technician opened the door and pulled me out, my eyes were about to pop out of my head and the horror was clearly written all over my face. That's when she told me we could have talked to each other the entire time – if I hadn't intended to nap!

When I had to have an MRI for this treatment and with this experience still fresh in my mind, I asked for something to take the edge off. I filled the prescription and was given three little white pills. I can't remember what they were, but they worked great. I was told to take one pill about an hour before my appointment, which would help me relax by the time I arrived. When I was changing into a gown, I thought, "I wonder why they gave me three. Maybe I should take another one just to make sure I'm good and relaxed. I don't want to be known as the woman who freaked out and went berserk having an MRI." I took a second pill and waited patiently for my turn.

My world mellowed at that point. Lazily, I followed the technician down the hall, staggering back and forth, two steps forward and one step back. When we got into the room for the MRI, I remember thinking the technician asked me to lie on my stomach on the table. Shouldn't my breast be face up? I was in no mood to argue, nor did I really care. (To this day, I couldn't even tell you if the equipment was open or closed.) The next thing I remember was feeling like my arms were two limp spaghetti noodles dangling over the sides of the table. I grinned, thinking I was just like the woman in the V8 commercial who was so tired her hands were dragging behind her as she walked through the front door of her home. I started laughing as I wondered how on earth I was going to get my long arms back into the sleeves of my shirt! Needless to say, I don't remember much more about that day – but it was the best and most stress-free MRI ever!

Lumpectomy or Mastectomy

TIP: **Do your homework, be proactive, and learn about your choices. If you are given the option of having either a lumpectomy or mastectomy, be confident your decision is the right one for you and your situation.**

Because my cancer was found early and was so small, I was fortunate to have several treatment options:

- I could have a lumpectomy followed by radiation treatments five days a week for approximately six weeks.
- I could choose to have a single mastectomy—only removing the breast with the cancer.
- I could choose a bilateral mastectomy, which involved removing both of my breasts.

The lumpectomy and mastectomy are two entirely different types of surgical procedures with different post-operative results and different recovery times.

If I chose to have a mastectomy, then there were two choices for reconstruction:

- Implanting temporary expanders at the time of the mastectomy. These would gradually be injected with a saline solution, which would slowly increase the size of the expanders (and my breasts) over a number of weeks. They would be removed some months later and replaced with artificial implants.
- Creating implants using skin, fat, and muscle taken from my abdomen. As I mentioned in chapter one, this procedure is called a TRAM, which is similar to having a tummy tuck, except the tissues that are removed are used to create the implants. Plus, a segment of muscle is also taken to provide the blood supply to keep the tissues alive.

Reconstruction with expanders and artificial implants provide a quicker recovery. Reconstruction from a TRAM requires a longer recovery because of the abdominal surgery.

My breast surgeon provided me the names of two plastic surgeons (and promised other referrals, if I wanted them). He suggested I ask each one what they recommended specifically for my situation.

Selecting a Plastic Surgeon

TIP: **Research, consult, and ask for recommendations of plastic surgeons that specialize in reconstructive surgery. Some may specialize in one particular procedure more than another. Do your homework!**

I took my breast surgeon's advice and scheduled consultations with two plastic surgeons. I was initially overwhelmed after meeting with the first one. While waiting in the examination room, I was shown a book with actual photos of women who had had mastectomies with various types of reconstruction. I started wondering if I had made the right decision in choosing to have a mastectomy and TRAM. I realized I needed to slow down and process everything I had learned before making a decision.

The second surgeon had been recommended by about half of the breast cancer survivors I had contacted. Once I met him, it was easy to understand why so many women chose him to do their TRAM reconstruction. He was personable and professional.

What I liked most was how he went into such great detail explaining how he would use my own tissues to form the breast implants, resulting in a more natural effect. He made sure I totally understood the "free TRAM" procedure, the recovery involved, and the anticipated outcome. Because I didn't have much excess stomach fat, he said I would have the option of having small artificial implants added about four months after the mastectomy. He likened having a bilateral mastectomy and TRAM to having breast implants plus a tummy tuck. My pink lemonade just got twice as sweet.

I also learned that the surgeon who treats you for the longest period of time while you are in the hospital is the admitting physician. By electing to have the abdominal TRAM, which required a longer hospital stay, my plastic surgeon would be my primary physician.

On my next visit to my breast surgeon, I told him which plastic surgeon and which reconstructive procedure I wanted to have. He supported my decision. I felt extremely fortunate to have a surgeon in whom I had 100% confidence and who encouraged me to be involved in the decisions.

Insurance Coverage for Reconstructive Surgery

TIP: **Contact your insurance company and learn exactly how much of the surgical expense they will cover, as well as what your co-pay and out-of-pocket expenses will be, including coverage for reconstruction.**

In 1997, a law was passed stating that insurance companies that cover mastectomies are required by law to cover the additional cost of breast reconstruction following a mastectomy.

To learn more, go to the website of the United States Department of Labor Employee Benefits Security Administration: http://www.dol.gov/dol/topic/health-plans/womens.htm.

Hospital Programs and Seminars

TIP: In your surgeon's office, ask for brochures about seminars, treatments, and support groups. Contact the breast center at your local hospital. Hospitals offer a number of programs that support breast cancer survivors. Non-profit organizations also offer additional programs.

During the first visit to my surgeon's office the morning after being diagnosed, I picked up a brochure about a "Breast Cancer Orientation" event scheduled for the following Monday night. I couldn't wait to attend and learn more from the hospital's perspective on what I could expect. My husband and daughter said they wanted to go with me, and I appreciated their interest and continued support.

There were only seven of us at the meeting: two other breast cancer survivors like myself, our three husbands, and my daughter, Lauren. The program lasted about an hour and covered several things I already knew and so many more I didn't know. I was so glad that I went.

One of the couples vanished as soon as it was over. I guessed she was still in the preliminary stages and needed private time to process what she was experiencing. The other couple had been sitting directly behind us. They stayed and introduced themselves. Debbie and I clicked immediately. We shared our similar situations.

After getting acquainted, Debbie looked at me and said, "Let's send our husbands home and go somewhere for coffee and talk." We did just that, choosing a nearby restaurant and requesting a table at the back, away from other patrons. We each spread our reports and research all over the table and compared our diagnoses and treatments. It was not long before the restaurant was packed. Every time a waiter or customer walked close to our table, we would both lean forward over our pictures and sketches and laugh like two little girls caught looking at nude pictures. It was during this time with Debbie that I made the final decision to have the mastectomy with TRAM reconstruction. What a blessing for me that Debbie and I had this opportunity to meet and discuss our situations.

We each had cancers similar in size and in our right breasts. We both were having bilateral mastectomies and abdominal TRAMS. Although we weren't using the same surgeons, we would be having our surgeries at the same hospital. Debbie's surgery was scheduled ten days before mine.

Looking at our watches, we couldn't believe we had been talking for almost three hours. During that time, we shared our thoughts and our concerns, knowing the other understood exactly what the other was feeling. Did I tell you we laughed? I know people were wondering what we were up to, especially if they had seen our nude pictures. After that, we had a bond as close as two peas in a pod. (This is Southern for "sisters.") We soon realized we had started a special friendship that was going to last a lifetime. I feel blessed and so fortunate that our paths crossed at the hospital that night. Every breast cancer survivor needs a "Debbie" like I have.

Choices

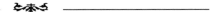

TIP: **You will be faced with making many decisions. The choices you make should be 100% yours and supported by your surgeon. Don't simply do what other people think you should do.**

After extensive research, talking with numerous breast cancer survivors, and having several surgical consultations, I met again with my breast surgeon to share the choices I had made.

I told him that I had definitely decided on having a bilateral mastectomy and TRAM reconstruction for the following reasons:

- At age 60, married, mother of three grown children and seven grandchildren, I was not concerned about losing my natural breasts. They were on the small side and had already served their purpose in nursing three children.
- I had strong support with my decision from my husband and my children.
- I knew I would have ongoing help from family and friends throughout my recuperation.
- By being self-employed, I would have the option of gradually returning to work at my own pace as I regained my strength and stamina.
- By having both breasts removed and reconstructed at the same time, my breasts would be symmetrical and balanced.
- In *my* mind, I didn't want to take a chance on cancer developing in my other breast some time in the future.

What a relief! I had total confidence in my decision, in my breast surgeon and in my plastic surgeon. I was ready to schedule my surgery, get it all behind me, and move on with living.

CHAPTER 3

Prior to Surgery

I have always enjoyed working on projects—the bigger the better. I love planning, organizing, researching, and implementing. During my years as a Girl Scout, I took the motto, "Be prepared," literally. "I believe in doing the very best you can do and avoid any regrets later."

My surgeons, their nurses and staff, and other breast cancer survivors were a tremendous help, but there were so many things I learned on my own. I was not experienced in having surgery or even being a patient in the hospital, other than when I had my babies (which I knew would not be quite the same as this), so this experience was all new to me.

I relied heavily on carrying my journal and a pencil with me at all times. Whenever I would brainstorm or random ideas would pop in my head, I would write them down. I tried to be creative and think of every possible scenario so I could ask questions and avoid any surprises.

Scheduling Surgery

TIP: **Being the first case of the day guarantees your surgery will happen on time. If you don't ask to be first, you may be put anywhere on the schedule and risk having your surgery delayed.**

I learned the hard way about the importance of choosing the time of day for surgery. My excisional biopsy was not scheduled until 11:00. I couldn't have anything to eat or drink after midnight the night before, so besides being hungry from not eating breakfast, I also missed my morning coffee. I saw it as a minor inconvenience … until my surgery was postponed for several hours until mid-afternoon.

The problem started when I developed a slight headache about noon. It gradually increased in intensity to the point that I couldn't concentrate on my Sudoku puzzles. With each passing hour, the headache became more severe. By the time they took me to the operating room for surgery, I had a full-blown migraine. We realized it was probably triggered by fasting and missing out on my morning cup of caffeine.

For several hours, the nurses gave me different pain medications before finally giving me morphine. After that, I really didn't care what time they operated on me!

I learned my lesson. When scheduling my mastectomy, I made sure I was the first patient of the morning. I also liked believing that the surgeons and all of the medical teams were fresh at the beginning of the day.

Action Plan

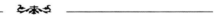

TIP: **Create a plan for yourself and your treatment. This gives you (and everyone else) confidence that you are in control.**

By choosing to have a bilateral mastectomy and reconstruction with a free abdominal TRAM, the first half of my treatment plan was underway. To execute the second half of my plan, I knew I needed all of the support I could get, so I decided to spread the word and tell everyone I knew. For many, this was the first they had heard of my diagnosis. I asked for their help in three ways.

First, I asked for prayers for strength for me, my family and friends, and expertise for my two surgical teams and the medical staff. The healing part was totally up to God.

Second, I asked friends to send me anything and everything that would make me laugh. They really came through on this. They sent me the most hilarious YouTube links, jokes, funny stories, and even books on humor.

And third, I asked for support in helping me decrease my stress. I realized that things that had once caused me stress were not really that big of a deal. I no longer allowed things to upset me or cause me to worry. I didn't accept any new responsibilities and I let go of many others.

Eliminate Stress

TIP: **Make a commitment that you will not allow other people or circumstances cause you to be stressed. Learn to let go of the less important obstacles and focus your attention only on the things that matter the most. Keep reminding yourself that not everything needs to be perfect. Don't be hard on yourself or on others, especially if they are trying to help you. Stress is a self-induced energy drain that affects you both mentally and physically.**

Whenever I felt myself get tense, I would stop and think, "Is there anything I can do to make the situation better?" If the answer was no, I would forget about it and move on.

It wasn't easy, but it was also not impossible to keep that commitment. In fact, Jim picked up on this technique and we became mellow together. It was a real bonus to a couple who had been married for almost 40 years.

Just sitting and having nothing to do used to be a major form of stress for me. I could always think of 101 things I could be doing other than sitting around and waiting, especially for appointments. Over the course of a few months, I spent countless hours sitting in waiting rooms or on exam tables.

I discovered that solving Sudoku puzzles was a great way to pass the time and exercise my brain. I even worked on them while lying on the gurney prior to my surgeries. I went through about five books during the first several months after being diagnosed.

To eliminate even more stress, I usually quit before I got to the "hard" sections. I always kept a book in my car and one in my purse, along with a pencil with a good eraser. (I now have an electronic version on my Blackberry.)

I tried to maintain my stress level, which I was able to control about 85% of the time. Whenever I would feel it creeping back again, I would refocus and repeat several mantras like:

- This too shall pass.
- Focus on solutions, not problems.
- Tomorrow is a new day and a fresh start.
- Worry does not solve problems.
- Things don't need to be perfect to be great.

Physical Fitness

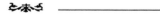

TIP: **The body heals faster when it is in good physical condition. With approval from your surgeon, start exercising today! It doesn't have to be high impact. Just start walking to get your blood circulating, your heart beating faster, and your lungs taking in more oxygen. What you do prior to surgery can have an impact on the speed of your recovery.**

Several months before being diagnosed, my daughters challenged me to compete in a sprint triathlon. What was I thinking? It was easy for them because they were in good shape and had competed in them before. Besides, they were more than 25 years younger than me!

Exercise had always been at the bottom of my priority list. I hated to sweat, feel pain, or be sore. Besides, I didn't like to exercise if it was too hot, too cold, too wet, too dry, too humid, too late, or too early.

Not wanting to be considered a wimp, I accepted their challenge and started "thinking" about my initial training.

As you can imagine, my plans for a new challenge changed from competing in a triathlon to having a bilateral mastectomy. With upcoming surgery, I was on a new mission. I suddenly felt the need to be in the best physical condition possible. Although I couldn't control having cancer, I knew that exercise was one area of my life I could control. When I asked my surgeons if it was okay for me to exercise prior to my surgery, they both agreed it would be good for me and gave me the "okay" to do what ever I felt like doing.

It was spring and the weather was absolutely beautiful. I started looking forward to my morning walks in our neighborhood. I loved walking early just as the sun was rising. It was a special time of the day when I could reflect, meditate, and mentally work on my game plan. Over time, I gradually worked on increasing my distance and decreasing my time. The day before my surgery, I walked three miles in 50 minutes! I thought that was good for a non-athlete.

Create a CaringBridge Website

TIP: CaringBridge is a free website service where you can set up your own web page to post your health related story and updates as well as receive comments from friends. It provides people with changing medical conditions a way to keep family and friends informed. The link is http://www.caringbridge.org.

A friend suggested I check into CaringBridge and set up a website so people could follow my progress without having to call and ask Jim. This relieved him from having to make so many phone calls and gave me a tremendous boost every time I read the notes friends posted in my guestbook.

The instructions for setting up a CaringBridge website page are easy to follow and the site offers a variety of templates. I chose one that had daffodils and was bright and cheery. I created my page the week before my mastectomy and sent an email to everyone I knew with the link and instructions on how to log on and stay updated on my progress.

I wish I had not selected the option requiring guests to create and use a password every time they logged on to my CaringBridge site. This confused and frustrated some of my non-technological friends. I later removed this option so friends were able to go directly to my home page as soon as they logged on.

I told friends if they wanted to receive an email notification automatically every time I posted a journal update, they could check the appropriate box on the journal page.

It was just as beneficial for me to have a place to share my thoughts as it was for friends to keep up with how I was doing. The link to my personal page is http://www.caringbridge.org/visit/marthalanier.

My site will remain active for as long as people read my updates and leave comments. I regularly log on and read the encouraging messages people have entered on my guestbook pages.

Point of Contact

TIP: **Ask a friend to be a point of contact to check on you, coordinate meals, run errands, drive you to appointments, walk your dog, help with your children, or provide any other help you might need. This is especially helpful if you live alone. Even if you have someone with you all of the time, this is a nice way to provide them with a backup and give others an opportunity to help.**

Fortunately, Jim was able to help me after I came home from the hospital. We definitely could have gotten by on his limited culinary skills, but the home-cooked meals delivered to our door each night for several weeks were something we both thoroughly enjoyed.

I am forever thankful to a neighbor who kept our entire neighborhood up to date on my progress. She coordinated who would bring meals and when.

Jim helped me in the morning and in the evening. He would have liked to have stayed with me all day, but I sent him back to work shortly after I came home from the hospital. Being independent, I enjoyed this quiet time of relaxing and doing things on my own and at my own pace.

Although friends offered to drive me to doctors' appointments, Jim jumped at the opportunity and enjoyed the responsibility of chauffeuring me until I was able to regain control of the wheel.

If you live alone, it is particularly important to have someone check on you daily to make sure you are okay and to bring you anything you may need.

Thank You Notes

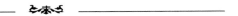

Before I went to the hospital, I bought several boxes of thank you cards and stamps. I put them in a canvas bag along with a notepad, where I kept a list of everyone who gave me flowers, brought dinners or gifts. Along with the addresses from my own address book, I also had my neighborhood and organization directories.

Although I had good intentions, I did not have the stamina or the mental sharpness to write the notes for quite some time after surgery (Don't worry; I cover memory loss in a later chapter). For weeks, I carried this little bag around with me from the recliner in the den to the glider on the porch to the floor next to my bed. It was some time before I felt like writing the first note. It helped having everything together at my fingertips and I soon found that writing several notes a day was therapeutic and something I enjoyed.

Personal Journal

I have a lifelong habit of keeping a personal journal. During my cancer journey, I realized how valuable keeping a record of my thoughts would be to me at the time as well as later.

About the time of my biopsy, I started writing faithfully every day. I even went back and added experiences that happened earlier in the year so I would have the entire journey documented. Since I knew Jim was on an emotional trip of his own, I suggested he keep a record of his thoughts too.

During the healing process, I realized how easy it was to forget many of the emotions and feelings I experienced. Now that so much time has passed, I am thankful I took the time to write down what I was feeling.

Reaching and Lifting

TIP: **Find a new location for things you use that are typically stored higher than your shoulder or on the floor. Buy items in smaller quantities so they are not heavier than a gallon of milk.**

I was told I could not raise my elbows higher than my shoulders for at least three weeks after surgery. At first I thought, "No problem." Then about a week before my surgery, I realized how many everyday items were out of my reach.

For several days, every time I reached up for something, I immediately found it a new home. This included things like cereal bowls, coffee mugs, glasses, shampoo, laundry detergent, towels, and extra rolls of paper towels, just to name a few.

It wasn't until after I returned home that I realized there were even more things I couldn't reach. I kept a list so Jim could help me when he came home. I later realized that for the most part, the only reason I wanted those things was because I couldn't reach them. I would think about something I had not used in months and suddenly decide I wanted it. Isn't it funny how our minds play games with us?

I was also told not to lift anything heavier than a full gallon of milk. This meant buying smaller containers for items such as detergent. I have a friend who bought a huge bag of cat litter and then realized after she got home from the hospital she couldn't lift it!

The hardest part for me was not being able to pick up my grandchildren. They just didn't seem to understand. Not to worry, I made up for it later!

Backrest Pillow Forms

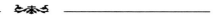

TIP: **Before you go to the hospital, plan how you will sleep once you come home. After having a mastectomy, my surgeon told me to sleep sitting up. Since my abdomen was so tight from the TRAM surgery, I also needed to sleep with my knees bent.**

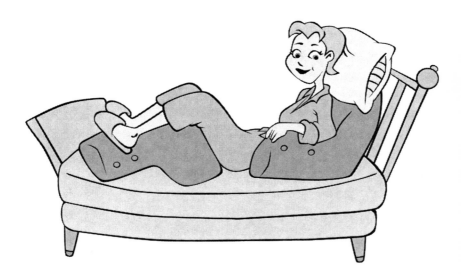

Since I didn't have a hospital bed at home, I had to come up with a creative way of sleeping at night that was as comfortable as possible. I remembered how in college I would use a backrest to lean on so I could read or study on my bed. We called it a "husband." It was a firm pillow with two arms extending from either side. It had literally been years since I had seen one of those, but I thought it was an ingenious idea. I knew I could solve my problem of sitting up while sleeping if I could just find one of those husband pillows. I was afraid regular pillows would slide and move around.

About a week before surgery, I found one at Target. I bought it and tried it out that night. Bingo! It worked great, especially if I propped other pillows on top of it for my head.

Then I realized that because of the abdominal surgery, I would need something to keep my knees bent while I slept. I bought another one, flipped it over so it was upside down, and placed it under my knees. This concept worked great! I was as comfortable as I could possibly be in my makeshift hospital bed.

Other options are to use triangular or wedge-shaped pillows. You can also stack several bed pillows under your knees.

For the first week or two after coming home from the hospital, I stayed in a recliner during the day. Although it was extremely comfortable, I found it took a great deal of effort to recline or push forward to get up out of the chair. My arms were weak and my pectoral muscles were sore. I also couldn't use my abdominal muscles to lower the footrest or sit up. At times, I floundered with my arms and legs in the air like a turtle stuck on his back until Jim came to my rescue.

Bed Height

TIP: **Adjust the height of your mattress. It is easier to get in and out of bed if the top of the mattress touches the backs of your knees when standing. If it is higher, you'll have to get up on your toes and slide onto the bed, causing you to be unsteady. If it is lower, you will have to bend forward and use your sore stomach muscles.**

The mattress on my bed is extremely high. In fact, I use a step stool every night to get up on it. I knew the height was going to be impossible to manage after surgery. I didn't want to risk slipping or falling off of the stool.

I backed my knees up to every bed in our house trying to find a mattress that was at just the right height. I felt like the little bear in the Goldilocks story! Although I had another bed I could sleep in, I wanted to be in my own bed, in my own room, with my adjoining bathroom. Once I found the right height, I came up with a solution.

First, I went to Home Depot and had six wood slats cut to fit the width of my bedframe. Next, I removed the mattress, box springs, and all of the slats. I put the box springs on the floor beneath the bed frame (I couldn't think of a better place to store a queen-sized box spring). Then I placed the new slats I had just bought—along with the original four—on the frame ridges. I then put my pillow-top mattress on top of the slats. Problem solved!

Since I could not really use my arms to pull myself up to get out of bed, I gently rolled to the outside, slid my feet off the edge of the mattress, and then leaned over the side of the bed. I found it was helpful if I concentrated on using my legs to do most of the work.

My bed stayed this way until I was about six weeks post-op, before I returned it to its original setup.

Sleepwear

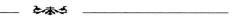

TIP: Remember that the clothing you decide to sleep in can't go on over your head, because you won't be able to raise your arms.

Wearing gowns was not an option because I could not easily get them over my head or my arms in the sleeve openings. If the neck was big enough, I could step into it and then pull it up. For the first week, I also needed fabric strong enough to pin my drainage bulbs to so they would be secure while I slept. This meant the fabric couldn't be too thin or flimsy.

Someone had given me the great idea of sleeping in nightshirts because they button up the front. The only problem was I really had a difficult time finding them. Not easily defeated, I went on a mission to the mall, determined to find at least one. You wouldn't believe some of the strange looks some of the younger salespeople gave me. You would have thought I had asked for something out of the 1800s.

You might find this hard to believe, but I found several at Victoria's Secret. They definitely were not what I considered sexy, but at that point being sexy wasn't my main priority. I admit I felt a little provocative with my new breasts, knowing my nightshirt was from Victoria's Secret–even if it was cotton with long sleeves and a high neck.

My daughter, Liz also went on a mission of her own and bought me another one. She made this one special by having my monogram sewn on the pocket.

Don't tell anyone, but after my tubes were removed and I didn't have to worry about pins, I discovered I was so much more comfortable not having anything touch my skin, so I just slept in the nude. Now *that* was comfortable and definitely daring!

Post-Op Clothes

TIP: **Because you will need to wear clothes that are comfortable once you are home from the hospital, plan ahead and find things that are loose and easy to take on and off.**

First things first. Because I knew I wouldn't be able to wear a bra for a while, my plastic surgeon's nurse suggested I buy several camisoles. They were really comfortable and came in a variety of colors. They were also great to wear under blouses. I had to make sure to buy them large enough to slip over my head and down past my shoulders without lifting my arms. If they were loose enough, I could then put my hands in each armhole and slide the straps across my shoulders. The first ones I bought didn't have the second layer of fabric with elastic beneath the bust line. I think I now have one of these in every color. To this day, I still enjoy wearing them.

Next, I bought loose blouses that could be left open or buttoned up the front. I wore them over my camisoles.

My abdomen was slightly swollen in the beginning so I definitely didn't want anything tight around my waist. I bought several pairs of slacks and capri pants with loose elastic waistbands or drawstrings. I was fortunate that my surgery was scheduled for the week after Memorial Day and I was able to take advantage of great holiday sales.

Wearing bright colors and comfortable clothes always helped me feel better. I never stayed in my gown and robe. I showered, dressed, and put on makeup every morning, even if I wasn't going anywhere and didn't expect company. I just considered this part of my recovery regimen.

24-Hour Comedy

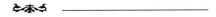

TIP: **At least several weeks prior to surgery, begin recording funny and entertaining TV shows and movies. That is also the time to buy videos and ask your friends if they have any DVDs you can borrow.**

I am not sure I totally understand why, but every post-mastectomy friend I have shares the same experience. It is impossible to sleep through the night for the first several months following the surgery. I would usually wake up about 2:00 or 3:00 a.m., stay awake for about an hour, fall back to sleep, and then wake up again long before it was time to get up.

Because my incisions were sore, it was virtually impossible to toss and turn. My choices were to lie awake staring at the ceiling or watch something entertaining on TV that didn't require too much concentration. I would turn on the TV, set the timer for 60 minutes, and occasionally fall back to sleep before it turned off. My standby for times when I couldn't sleep was watching *America's Funniest Home Videos* and reruns of comedy shows like *I Love Lucy, Three's Company*, and *Friends*.

If I was really bored during the day, I would watch videos or log onto my laptop computer and laugh hysterically at some of the YouTube links my friends had sent me.

I realized it made sense that laughing helped me breathe deeper, which in turn sent more oxygen through my bloodstream to help with the healing process. As we generally can only focus on one thing at a time, it is harder to experience pain while we are laughing. I am a firm believer that laughter really is the best medicine.

Special Treats

TIP: **Take the time to do special things for yourself. Make sure they are fun and enjoyable.**

The day before my surgery, I scheduled a manicure and a pedicure. Because of the abdominal surgery with the TRAM, I knew it would likely be several weeks before I could lean over and reach my toes.

I have had many manicures and pedicures in the past, but I created the image in my mind that this particular one was an extra-special treat. It was amazing how I felt more relaxed and savored every minute.

There were several times before surgery when Jim and I would plan an extra-special date night and go out for dinner and a movie. Even my shopping excursions, reorganizing my home, and just about everything else was done with the purpose of making it special. That one thing helped me maintain a positive attitude.

CHAPTER 4

Pre-Operative Preparation and Packing

You would have thought I was planning a trip around the world, or that if I forgot something, I would just have to do without ... as if Jim couldn't bring it to me from home or buy it at the nearby mall. Besides, what could I possibly need or want during my hospital stay?

Sentinel Node Mapping

TIP: **There is no preparation involved on your part for the sentinel node mapping other than showing up. Don't forget to take something to read or do, such as a Sudoku book in case you have a long wait.**

Sentinel node mapping is a procedure that identifies the lymph nodes located closest to the cancer site. My procedure was done as an outpatient at the hospital. Since my surgery was first on the schedule, the mapping had to be done late in the afternoon on the day before. The mapping allows the surgeon to locate and remove the lymph node closest to the cancer. During the surgery, it would be sent to pathology to determine if it contained cancer cells.

The x-ray technician numbed the skin near my biopsy incision. All I felt was a slight pinch. After about 15 minutes, he returned to give me the radioactive injection necessary to identify the sentinel node. I closed my eyes and held my breath, anticipating that I wasn't going to enjoy this procedure. I asked how long it would take to give me the injection and to please warn me before he did it. He chuckled and said, "I'm already finished."

I felt fine after getting the injection and offered to walk rather than ride in a wheelchair to the nuclear medicine department. I was told rather firmly that I was *required* to be pushed in a wheelchair. That was the first time I actually felt like a patient.

I was pushed down long hallways, took a trip on several elevators, and pushed down more hallways. We turned a corner and I noticed the walls were decorated with bright fluorescent yellow signs with warnings that read, "CAUTION—Nuclear Medicine."

I was positioned on a special table where a huge piece of equipment hovered only inches above me. Because the sides were open, I managed to ward off a claustrophobic panic attack. After what seemed like an eternity, the technician removed the overhead equipment, popped the top off of his black magic marker, and proceeded to draw a treasure map all across my right breast and armpit. Thank goodness I shaved that morning. How embarrassing would it have been if I hadn't?

Before I left, I was threatened with my life … well, not really, but I had to promise I would not attempt to wash off his artwork when I showered the next morning.

I was glad I had an escort on my return trip because there was no way I could have remembered how to get back to where we had started. Relieved that it was over, I got dressed and was released. Later that evening, Jim teased me that I glowed in the dark (He was kidding, of course).

'Twas the Night Before Surgery

—————————— 乙末彡 ——————————

TIP: **If you are having an abdominal TRAM and have been given a laxative to take the day before, don't wait until too late in the day to take it. Trust me --- I learned this the hard way!**

I wish someone had told me to take my laxative earlier in the afternoon on the day before my surgery. After dinner, I became distracted when I started packing. It was almost 8:00 before I realized I had not taken the laxative.

I chased it with a bottle of water, finished packing and then drank a second bottle of water, thinking it would generate some activity. By midnight, things were *still* calm and quiet. Finally, I decided to go to bed and let nature do its thing while I slept. I had to get up in four short hours so we could get to the hospital by 5:00 a.m., my required check-in time.

My alarm went off at 4:00. The laxative waited until I had one foot in the shower before hitting me. After five attempts, I finally managed to take the fastest shower of my life, throw on some clothes and get in the car just as Jim was pulling out of the driveway. I actually thought he was going to leave without me! He kept mumbling that we were going to be late. In my mellow, non-stressed state, I gave him a smile and said, "Well, I'd like to see them start without me!"

We made it down two streets and as far as our neighborhood pool before nature called again. Thank goodness, the restroom door was not locked. I got back in the car and ten minutes later yelled for Jim to stop again. This time we made it to a convenience store and gas station. How apropos!

By this time, Jim was calculating that with the frequency of my pit stops, we should arrive at the hospital about lunchtime; so much for his destressing. We finally arrived at the hospital, but halfway through the admitting process, I interrupted the nurse, held up my finger and said, "Hold that thought, I'll be right back!"

Bathrobe and Bedroom Slippers

TIP: Because of the size of the drainage bulbs, a wrap-around bathrobe is the only kind that will fit. Slippers are easy to get on and off. Additionally, they make you feel a little more stylish than when wearing the hospital socks with the skid-proof grips.

When packing, I planned on taking my long, soft, fluffy bathrobe that zipped up the front. It was the warmest and most comfortable robe I had. I packed it because I thought it would be easy to get on and off.

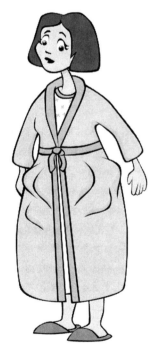

At the last minute, I decided it was taking up too much room, so I replaced it with my long silky wrap-around robe. I didn't know at that time that I would have six drainage tubes with grenade-sized bulbs at the end of each one! There was no way possible my zippered robe would have worked. In fact, the wrap-around robe barely met in the front. At least it did the job! I felt as big around as the Pillsbury doughboy.

The hospital gave me skid-proof socks to keep me from slipping, but because my arms were weak and my feet were essentially out of reach, it was hard to get them on and off. I found it was much easier to slide my feet into my own slippers, plus they also matched my robe. My theory is that when you look good, you naturally feel good!

All of the Necessities

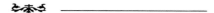

TIP: Bring your own toiletries with you to the hospital, even though the basics are generally provided.

Although the hospital provided the basic necessities, they weren't the same as those I used at home. I was really thankful I had my own toothbrush, toothpaste, shampoo, conditioner, soap, and definitely my makeup. I was so glad I remembered to pack my makeup mirror, too.

I decided to leave my razor and shaving cream at home, knowing clean-shaven legs would not be high on my priority list; plus, I figured I wouldn't be able to reach them for a while anyway. I felt better knowing I had all of the basics I would possibly need. Besides, I wasn't going to be in the hospital that long.

Family Photos

TIP: Bringing your favorite photos from home will give you a comforting and warm feeling of love and support, even when your friends and family are not there with you.

I found an 11" x 14" Lucite frame several days before my surgery. To help my hospital room feel more like home, I made a collage using some of my favorite family pictures. I included a special photo of Jim, pictures of our three children and their spouses, and photos of our seven precious grandchildren. Jim placed the frame in a prominent spot on one of the shelves in the corner of my room where I could easily see it from my bed.

My nurses, doctors, and everyone who came to see me also enjoyed seeing the photos. They asked me who everyone was, who belonged to whom, and all about my children and grandchildren. At times when I was alone, I felt like my family was all right there with me.

Cell Phone and Charger

TIP: An easy way to receive calls and stay in touch with family and friends is with your cell phone. (Don't forget to bring your charger!)

I quickly realized that using my cell phone was so much easier than trying to answer the hospital phone. Besides, I had every phone number or email address I could possibly need stored in my Blackberry. I thoroughly enjoyed making and receiving calls. When I got tired and wanted to rest, I just put it on vibrate or turned it off.

I found it extremely difficult to reach and answer the hospital phone by my bed. We even moved it from the bedside table to the tray stand. For me, it was easier to pick up the receiver and answer the phone if it was hung up backwards. The only problem was the nurses kept turning it back around every time they came in my room!

Humor in the Hospital

TIP: Since humor is said to be the best medicine, use it not only to help with your healing, but also lift the spirits of everyone around you.

My friends went all out sending me jokes and funny stories. Before my surgery, I decided to print several pages of my favorites and take them with me, along with some I thought the nurses would enjoy.

We taped a page or two to the wall behind my bed. I wanted my nurses to be happy and in good moods when they came in to take care of me. Once I started walking the halls, I decided to take some of them to the nurses' station so all of the nurses could enjoy them.

Now that I think about it, an even better idea would have been to tape the jokes and funny stories on the outside of the door of my room. That way, all of the nurses and the other patients walking the halls could also enjoy them and have a good laugh too.

Chapter 5

In the Hospital

When I was seven, I had my tonsils removed and stayed just one night in the hospital. I don't remember anything other than eating popsicles and ice cream. When each of my children were born, I stayed only two nights in the hospital and don't remember anything other than fulfilling my dream of being a mom and learning about new babies.

This time I knew my hospital stay would be totally different. The experience was going to be new and unfamiliar and I wasn't sure what to expect. One important lesson I have learned since becoming a business owner is not to try to be an expert at everything, just at what you do best. It is more important to get help and rely on people who are trained and skilled in what they know and do.

I knew I was going to be in an excellent hospital on a surgical floor with nurses who specialized in caring for post-mastectomy patients. In my mind, I knew I was in the best place possible. Before I was admitted, I decided I was going to move into my hospital room both physically and mentally. I planned on taking advantage of the expertise of those who would be taking care of me. I knew they would be doing their part to help me get better and it was my responsibility to do my part. Together we would be a great team.

Anesthesia

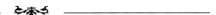

TIP: Prior to surgery, ask your anesthesiologist to do whatever he or she can do to keep you from feeling nauseated when you wake up – a potential side effect of anesthesia.

Although I had never experienced nausea after having surgery, this was one time I definitely wanted to make sure it didn't happen, especially after the abdominal TRAM procedure.

I discussed my concern with the anesthesiologist when she met with me prior to my surgery. She reassured me I had nothing to worry about.

Whatever the anesthesiologist gave me worked! I never felt nauseated. In fact, I even woke up feeling a little hungry, but truthfully that was not unusual for me!

Home Away From Home

TIP: Home is where the heart is. Mentally move into your hospital room, knowing it is where you will receive excellent care for the next several days.

I told myself how fortunate I was to be in such a wonderful hospital and on a surgical floor where I knew I would receive the best possible care from the most experienced, well trained, and caring nurses, technicians, and staff.

Mentally, I moved into my room and was a patient in every sense. I was relieved that I really didn't have to worry about anything but healing and getting better. I had total confidence in my doctors, my nurses, and the staff. I never thought about what time I needed to take my medicine or how often. I knew they would adhere to a strict schedule when it came to changing my IV or milking my drains. I even had excellent help in taking showers. My sheets were changed first thing each morning and my floor was swept clean daily.

All of that gave me the opportunity to focus my efforts on feeling better and getting well. The entire staff treated me royally during my hospital stay. I felt like it was truly my home away from home.

Surgical Dressings and Baby Blankets

TIP: **Don't be surprised at any of the post-operative procedures. Different surgeons have different ways of dressing your incisions.**

I was shocked and somewhat surprised when I first looked down and saw a baby blanket from the hospital nursery neatly folded across my chest. Still groggy, I had a flashback to the conversation when Jim asked if I was pregnant. I was trying to remember if I actually had a mastectomy or if I was getting ready to nurse a newborn.

I don't think the pale blue, pink, and white-striped baby blankets have changed since my children were born over 35 years ago. I was relieved when a nurse explained the blanket was to keep my new breasts warm, not in preparation to cuddle a baby.

The First Sneak Peek

TIP: **If you have a TRAM, realize that you will go to sleep on the operating table with breasts, and you will wake up in the recovery room with breasts.**

Boy was I surprised when I took a look at my surgical sites for the first time. I expected to see huge gauze bandages covering both my chest

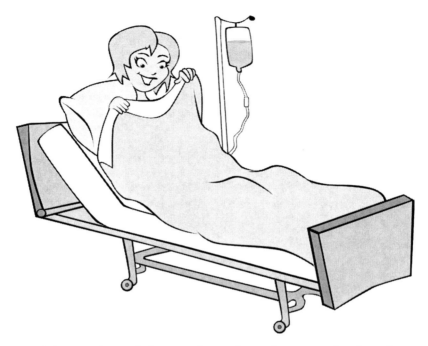

and abdomen. Instead, I remember only seeing several strips of paper tape on my new breasts and a strip across my abdomen.

First, I remember looking down at my chest. I saw two shapely breasts. Obviously, there were bruises and indications that I'd had major surgery, but it was nothing at all like I had expected. The incisions were clean and tight and covered with a thin piece of paper tape. And my new breasts were even larger than my original ones!

Next, I looked at my stomach. My TRAM incision was covered with a piece of paper tape that extended from one hipbone to the other all the way across my lower abdomen. My new belly button was as pretty as a picture. This may be a slight exaggeration, but trust me, it all looked better than I had imagined.

At first, I had my doubts about the strength and effectiveness of the skimpy little paper tape covering my incisions, especially on my lower abdomen. My immediate thought was, "I'm being held together with paper tape! What happens when I sneeze? If they had asked me, I would have suggested they use duct tape."

The nurses assured me that my surgeon had used plenty of stitches beneath my skin to hold my incisions tightly together. The paper tape was there to keep the incision scar from stretching. What a relief!(I'll talk more about the magic of paper tape a little later.)

In my opinion, the reconstructive surgery that they perform today following a mastectomy is an absolute miracle.

First Night

TIP: **Be prepared for nurses to come in your room every 30 minutes for the first 24 hours. They will check to see there is a good blood supply to the grafted tissues.**

My daughter, Lauren stayed the first night with me to be my advocate and to help make any major decisions should it be necessary. We knew the nurses would be checking on me every 30 minutes to make sure the implanted grafts stayed warm and had good circulation.

I remember sometime in the middle of the night both of us bursting out laughing at all of the weird and unusual noises we were hearing in the room. There was the continuous rhythm of the machine measuring my blood pressure. I had electronic booties on my feet that mechanically expanded and contracted to keep the circulation flowing in my legs. There was the beeping sound when my IV bag was ready to be changed.

I had the greatest peace of mind knowing that I was being carefully monitored. I especially liked when my nurses came in to check on me. They were all friendly, gentle, and reassuring.

Two of my close friends also offered to stay overnight with me. Jean stayed the second night after my surgery just in case I needed help during the night. I declined at first because I didn't want her to have to stay awake all night, but after a little thought, I accepted her offer. I slept peacefully and didn't encounter any problems. I called Marcia the next morning and told her I didn't feel it was necessary for her to come the next night and watch me sleep. Besides, it would be much more fun if she came during the day so we could talk and visit.

Drainage Tubes

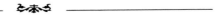

TIP: **When you wake up from surgery, don't be surprised to discover long thin tubes leading from your incisions down to grenade-shaped bulbs. Their purpose is to drain fluid that accumulates at the surgical sites. Other than making you feel like a cow at milking time, they are painless.**

This was the first time I had ever had drainage tubes. There were six: one on either side of each of my breasts and one at each end of my abdominal incision. I couldn't decide if I felt more like a dairy cow or an octopus with tentacles (except I only had six tubes, not eight)!

I had read in my pre-op information that I would have tubes and they would have to be "milked," but I had no idea what this meant. "Milking" is a fancy way of saying, "draining the excess fluid from the incision sites." The excess fluid is pushed gently through each tube and into a bulb at the other end. The fluid is then poured out of the bulbs into a small plastic cup where it is measured.

Once the amount of fluid that is drained from each bulb decreases below a specific amount in a 24 hour period, the doctor or nurse removes the tubes. Three of mine were removed before I left the hospital and the other three were removed during follow-up office visits.

While I was in the hospital, my drains were milked every four hours around the clock. During the night, I would often relax, lie still, and not say anything while the nurses did their work.

Pain Meds

꿏꿏꿏

TIP: **When your nurse tells you it is time to take your meds ... take them! This is one time you want to stay ahead of the pain before you have a chance to experience it.**

I realized this was not the time to prove how tough I was or how well I could tolerate pain. We all already know how strong women are! By taking my pain meds on time, I knew they would help me feel more like moving around. The more I moved around and walked, the better I would feel in the long run. Each day was easier than the day before.

Important note: if I waited about 20 minutes *after* taking my pain meds to get out of bed, shower, or walk, I realized that moving around was much easier and more comfortable. Throughout the entire day, I planned my activities around my pain management schedule, and it worked beautifully.

To keep from feeling nauseated, I made sure to have something in my stomach first. I found graham crackers tasted better and were easier to swallow than Saltines, which always seemed to stick to the roof of my mouth.

On my frequent walks, I liked going to the snack room down by the nurses' station and stocking up on crackers, apple juice, and crushed ice. I enjoyed having them for an afternoon snack; plus, it gave me an excuse to walk.

Stool Softeners

> **TIP:** Pain medication is great for relieving your pain, but works quite the opposite for relieving your bowels. You will probably want to request taking a stool softener.

In spite of my "colon cleansing" on the way to the hospital, I started asking for a stool softener the first day after surgery, since one of the side effects of taking narcotics is constipation. The thought of putting unnecessary strain on my fresh abdominal incision scared me. I did not yet have the urge to go, but I didn't want to wait until I needed to apply pressure. Initially, I was not concerned because I was not eating or exercising that much.

Although I was fortunate not to experience much pain in my abdomen, I was surprised at how tight it felt. I was very protective of my abdominal incision.

My surgeon prescribed daily doses of Colase—a gentle stool softener—along with my other meds. By the time my appetite returned, I had taken enough Colase that I definitely didn't have a problem.

Personal Hygiene and Makeup

> **TIP:** Nothing feels better than brushing your teeth, washing your face, and putting on make-up, even if it is just a little blush and lipstick or gloss. It will give you a boost that will jumpstart your day.

The nurses wasted no time getting me up and out of bed the first morning following my surgery. After brushing my teeth and washing my face, it felt great to put on a fresh hospital gown and get back into a bed with clean sheets. The nurses helped me the entire time. I didn't have to worry about a thing.

I remember how wonderful it felt to get back into my typical morning routine of washing my face and brushing my teeth. Putting on make-up also made me feel so much better, not to mention that I'm sure people probably thought I looked better, too. Although I have had short hair for years, I had it cut extra short several days prior to my surgery so it would be low-maintenance for at least several weeks.

Warm Showers

TIP: If your doctor has given you the go-ahead to shower, think of it as a mini-spa treatment and enjoy!

On the second morning, I was both surprised and thrilled when the nurses told me I could shower and wash my hair! Although it took some effort at first, I knew how much better I was going to feel afterward.

I was given a pair of stretch maternity underwear with the crotch cut out. It covered my breasts like a halter and provided something to pin my drainage bulbs onto so they didn't dangle.

I must admit I was relieved to see there was even a chair in the tub for me to sit on. I was able to lean forward and rest my elbows on my knees to wash my hair.

I thoroughly enjoyed being in the shower and remained there for the longest time, just relaxing and enjoying the warm, soothing water. Eventually I heard a knock on the bathroom door and a voice telling me I was going to shrivel up like a prune if I didn't get out. They all had fun teasing me about my marathon showers and shriveled skin.

With my short hair, there was no need to worry about styling it so I just let it air dry. Once I was back in bed, I propped up with about six pillows and nestled into my clean, fresh sheets. Although I was exhausted, I felt so much better and was ready for visitors or whatever the day would bring.

Daily Walks

On the morning following surgery, I was greeted with a team of nurses and medical technicians. My catheter was removed (what a relief!), and then was told they were there to change my linens and fluff my pillows. Northside Hospital was beginning to sound like a five-star

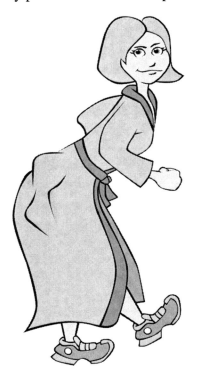

hotel. I soon realized this was really a nice way of saying, "It is time to get your bod out of bed and start walking." At first, I was nervous about standing up because of the abdominal surgery from the TRAM. This is often painful for some women, whether it is from having a basic tummy tuck or TRAM surgery.

Once I stood up, the only part of me that was vertical was from the waist down. I was a slow-moving right angle. I appeared as if I was looking for a lost contact lens. It was slow going, but at least I was moving on my own.

Once I was back in bed, I felt like I had achieved a major accomplishment by walking myself to the bathroom and back. I knew it could only get easier.

Getting out of bed to walk, move around and even sit in a chair helped clear my lungs, improve my blood flow and increase my stamina. Within a day or two, I was walking all over the surgical floor ... still bent forward. But at least I was moving.

Thank Your Nurses

———————————— ᤈᤁᤀ ————————————

TIP: "Thank you" is one of the most powerful phrases I know. It is not enough for people to assume we are pleased with their service or that they are just doing their job. Show your nurses how much you appreciate all they do for you.

I had been told that the nurses on the third floor of Northside Hospital who take care of hysterectomy and mastectomy patients were absolutely the most caring and skilled team. I learned firsthand how true this was. They all knew exactly how to meet my needs as well as provide the specific care my surgeon required. I had total confidence in each of them and valued how kind and thoughtful they were. I referred to them as my "nurse angels".

My sister gave me the idea of giving each shift of nurses a box of candy. Before I was discharged, Jim brought me three big boxes of gourmet chocolates, each with a big bow and a funny thank you card. It was so much fun surprising them!

CHAPTER 6

Post-Operative at Home

Because I was comfortable in my hospital room and confident with the care I received, I really wasn't all that excited about coming home. I was leaving my five-star accommodations where my sheets were changed daily, my pillows fluffed, the floor mopped, the bathroom cleaned, meals prepared, my incisions checked, my meds given to me on time, and all of my questions answered around the clock. I felt safe and secure and didn't have anything to worry about other than taking my daily walks, resting, focusing on feeling better, and regaining my strength.

To say I was nervous about leaving the safety and security of the hospital was an understatement. I just didn't have the confidence, nor did I want to accept the new responsibility of monitoring my pain meds and antibiotic, caring for my tubes and doing any of the unforeseen things that I might not know how to handle. Jim, on the other hand, was anxious to have me back home.

After the long drive home and getting back into my familiar surroundings, it didn't take long to start my new routine. Within an hour of settling into my recliner and surrounding myself with my hospital pillows, Jim and I talked and shared our feelings. He was then able to understand how he could support and reassure me and let me do things at my own pace. He shared his feelings, and for the first time I realized from his perspective what he had been experiencing. We had a new respect for each other and our emotions. He helped me feel safe, yet he gave me the freedom to be back in control. I enjoyed having him help me and I really was glad to be home again.

First Two Weeks Post-Op

———————————— ﴿﷽﴾ ————————————

TIP: **The first 14 days following surgery can be the most important when it comes to the speed of your recovery. Take things slow and easy for the first two weeks.**

Knowing that I am extremely active and enjoy life at a fast pace, my breast surgeon's scrub nurse looked me right in the eye and said just before I was discharged from the hospital, "If you will slow down and totally take it easy for the first 14 days following your surgery, you will be amazed at how much faster you will recover. Don't do much more than eat, sleep, and keep up with your walking."

Throughout the entire process, slowing down was by far the hardest thing for me to do. First, I gave myself permission to take it easy and allow my body to heal—all guilt free. Next, I convinced myself that this was not the time to prove to the world how strong or independent I was. So I propped up my feet, took frequent power naps, asked for help if I wanted something, and let others enjoy doing things for me.

By the morning of the 15th day I was rested and ready! There was no stopping me now! I was feeling fabulous and ready to push myself a little more and see what I felt like doing. Gradually I was able to build my strength and increase my stamina.

Accept Help

———————————— ﴿﷽﴾ ————————————

TIP: **Swallow your pride (and your stubbornness) and don't hold back when it comes to asking for help. At the same time, you won't be depriving friends of the satisfaction of enjoying the feeling that they are needed.**

It was a real reality check when I realized I was not the only person experiencing my diagnosis of breast cancer. It was not just about me. My family and friends were affected as well – just in a different way. Friends often offered to help, but had no idea what to do. I realized I could help them deal with my having cancer by allowing them to help me.

If someone offered to do something for me, I graciously accepted. I even tried to have responses ready when someone offered, but didn't know what I needed. I tried to be prepared and help them with suggestions.

An ideal comment was, "Thank you for offering. Dinner one night would be wonderful. Wednesday or Friday has not been claimed this week, or any night next week would be great."

I also knew that if there was something specific for which I did need help, I could always call a friend and just ask. Friends like to be needed. Who doesn't? Asking for and accepting help is a sign of strength, not weakness.

Medication Log

TIP: Create a system so you can record each time you take your pain medication, antibiotic, laxative, or other medications.

With my memory not operating at full capacity, I found it not only helpful, but a necessity, to keep a log with the name of each medication and the last time I took each of them. I couldn't remember when I was supposed to take what. To add to the confusion, at times I was sleeping during the day and staying awake at night. Some medications I took only once a day, some twice, and others every four hours. Rarely did they ever seem to coincide with each other.

Because I took my antibiotic every 12 hours, I used the alarm on my cell phone as a reminder each morning and each night. Pain meds were easier to monitor since I usually began watching the clock and anticipating how long it would be before I could take the next one.

Pain Management

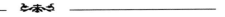

TIP: **You definitely want to manage the pain, but there are alternatives to the narcotics prescribed for you in the hospital. Talk to your surgeon about other options.**

Although I was pain free when taking the heavy drugs, I didn't like the strange way they made me feel. The day I came home from the hospital, I stopped taking the power drugs and switched to the over-the-counter pain medications my surgeon suggested.

I was fortunate that the only real discomfort I experienced was a burning sensation across my chest extending from one armpit over to the other. I was told this was a result of my nerves healing. This lasted for several weeks and gradually decreased in intensity each day. Although my abdomen was extremely tight for several weeks, I never really experienced much pain there. In talking with other "breast friends," they said their experience was just the opposite. They had more discomfort from their abdominal incision and less from their mastectomy. As I have said before, although our surgeries may be similar, our experiences are totally different. All women respond differently to the pain and healing.

I quickly realized that I could relieve some of the discomfort by taking warm showers. Another way was not wearing a blouse or top so that nothing touched my skin. The only problem with this was I just couldn't go around nude from the waist up all the time. That was when lightweight and loose blouses came in handy ... well, at least they beat the alternative!

Milking at Home

TIP: **You will be sent home from the hospital with all of the milking supplies you will need and detailed instructions on what to do. The good news is the tubes are not permanent. My favorite quote is, "This too shall pass." So will your tubes.**

After coming home, my surgeon said I only had to milk my remaining tubes three times during the day. Ask your surgeon how often you should milk yours.

Previously, I mentioned I am somewhat of a control freak. With this in mind, I was determined to take care of my tubes myself. I'm sure Jim would have done a great job, but this was something I wanted to do. Milking my tubes was not uncomfortable or painful, just something that was a necessary part of the healing process.

First, I put everything I needed on the counter in the bathroom. I always took my time and followed the procedures exactly as they were outlined. I kept all of my supplies in the plastic container they gave me in the hospital. I made sure I had the log sheet and a pen, alcohol wipes, and the small measuring cup handy.

After I washed my hands, I gently held each tube with my forefinger and thumb where it was close to my skin. With my other hand, I placed the sterile alcohol pad around the tube and squeezed the fluid down into the bulb at the end. I repeated this several times until the tube was empty. I then opened the bulb cap and poured the fluid into a small plastic measuring cup so I could measure it. With the top still off, I tightly rolled and squeezed the bulb to push out all of the air, replaced the cap, and pinned it back onto my shirt. I repeated this procedure with each tube and recorded the drained amount on my log, rinsed the cup and put everything back in my plastic container.

Once the amount of fluid from each bulb decreased below the amount specified by my surgeon, I scheduled an office visit so the doctor or his nurse could remove the drain.

Drainage Bulbs

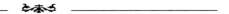

TIP: **Attaching your drainage bulbs to your clothing is important for both safety and comfort.**

During the day, I pinned the drainage bulbs to the underside of my shirt just above my waist. This way, I was not taking a risk sitting on them or having them dangle below my shirt line. (This is not cool when you have company or are going to see your doctor!)

At night, I soon realized that if the bulbs were pinned on the outside of the front of my nightshirt, I was more comfortable lying in bed and sleeping. I was also less likely to lie on top of one of them.

Warning! If you pin the bulbs on the outside of your clothes, be extra careful not to let the tubes get caught on doorknobs or drawer pulls. I feel the need to mention this because one time I turned quickly and came so close to getting hung on a drawer pull in the bathroom. I didn't want to think about the consequences if this had happened. I only did it once and realized it just in time. Needless to say, it made a lasting impression.

While showering in the hospital, I pinned the bulbs onto the mesh halter they gave me. Because it was so loose, I was always nervous it might slide down. Several days after being home, I found a fabric lanyard. I put it around my neck and pinned the bulbs to it. Bingo! It felt secure and I was confident the bulbs were not going to drop.

Power Naps

—————————————— ≿★≾ ——————————————

TIP: **One of the best ways for your body to heal is by resting. Give yourself permission to take naps – totally guilt free. Just make sure they are not too late in the afternoon.**

Before having surgery I used to feel guilty even thinking about closing my eyes for a quick power nap in the middle of the afternoon. But once I realized that resting my body and mind was a necessary step in the healing process, I not only gave in to the idea, but started looking forward to them every day after lunch.

This was great for the first few weeks. When I asked my surgeon for a prescription to help me sleep, he suggested that perhaps it was time for me to eliminate my naps. At least they were fun while they lasted!

Therapeutic Showers

—————————————— ≿★≾ ——————————————

TIP: **Warm showers can provide soothing, therapeutic, and healing results. Take them as often as you wish (with your doctor's approval, of course)!**

My surgeon confirmed I could continue my showers after coming home, as long as I didn't let the water hit directly on my incisions. I definitely could not have a tub bath until all my incisions had healed and the doctor said it was okay.

To receive the maximum benefit from my warm showers, I frequently stayed in there for 15 to 20 minutes. Just standing there letting the warm water splash on my back, neck, and shoulders was my ultimate form of relaxation. This soon became something I looked forward to every morning and just before going to sleep at night. This was my special personal time when I could totally relax. It was extremely effective in relaxing my muscles and helping me fall asleep.

In spite of being on water restrictions all summer due to a drought, I never gave a second thought to taking my marathon showers. After all, I considered them essential to my recovery.

Rebuilding Stamina

TIP: Once you are home, increase your exercise to increase your stamina.

Although I thoroughly enjoyed the slower pace and downtime in the beginning of my recovery, it wasn't long before I became anxious for some activity. After coming home, I enjoyed going outside in the morning while it was still cool and then going back out again in the evening after the sun had gone down. Often I would sit in a chair in our driveway, relaxing and breathing the fresh air. The change in scenery was a welcome relief. I especially liked it when neighbors would see me and stop for a visit.

At first, I walked up and down our driveway, gradually increasing the distance. I particularly remember one morning several days after coming home. I walked out to our mailbox to check on the petunias I had planted the weekend before my surgery. They were all alive and healthy. New buds were already popping out. Some of the original blooms were limp and needed to be picked.

I had the urge to squat down, but quickly realized that was not an option. If I was able to get down, I knew I would have to stay there until someone drove by and offered to help me back up. In our quiet neighborhood, I could be down for hours.

All of a sudden, I got a great idea! If I slipped off my sandal, I could prune them with my toes. Since I was a little girl, I have been known for having the ability to pick up just about anything with my toes. I always considered this a unique talent. As women, we can be resourceful when we need to be! About 20 minutes later, my flowerbed was once again vibrant with bright colors and the dead blooms were scattered and hidden throughout the bed.

That wasn't my only foray into being creative. One night after seeing me walk through our family room and up and down our stairs repeatedly, Jim asked if he could help me find whatever I had lost. I said, "No thanks, I have a new exercise route and I'm just extending my laps!" I didn't have to do that for long before my surgeon gave me the go-ahead to begin walking again throughout our neighborhood and later on the treadmill.

Paper Tape

TIP: **Paper tape is the best-kept secret when it comes to minimizing the size of incision scars. With your doctor's permission, use it to help keep the scar tissue from stretching as it heals.**

When I was discharged from the hospital, I was sent home with a supply of paper tape. I was instructed to continue putting it over my incisions until I was told to stop. The tape I used was one-inch wide.

Before each of my showers, I would press my fingers along both the top and bottom edges of the full length of each strip of the tape. This was to eliminate any potential air pockets and prevent moisture from getting trapped beneath the adhesive.

I changed the tape once each week and did this for about three months, which was probably longer than necessary. This could very well be why each of my incisions is now barely visible; only a hint of a fine, thin line remains. Although I don't plan on wearing a bikini, if I did, you wouldn't notice my scar. (My grown children will probably have heart failure at the thought of that picture!)

BONUS TIP: I found that paper tape is also great for protecting blisters! After walking 20 miles on the first day of the Atlanta 2-Day Walk for Breast Cancer, I developed two blisters—one on each foot. I knew from showering after surgery that moisture or, in this case, sweat, does not affect paper tape. Since I had put a roll of paper tape in my fanny pack before the walk, I tried wrapping the tape over my blisters and across several other problem spots. It worked great and I was able not only to wear my shoes the next day, but also to finish the last ten miles of the walk! In fact, I continued to use the paper tape until my blisters healed.

Pillows

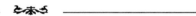

TIP: **Although hospital pillows are a standard size, they are relatively thin and easy to fold, roll, and stack for added comfort when sleeping and sitting. Ask if you can take yours home from the hospital.**

I could not believe how many bed pillows they gave me to use at the hospital. My bed looked like one huge cotton ball! They were the perfect answer in helping me find comfortable positions for sleeping and propping myself up in bed and even sitting in a chair. They fit in standard-size cases, yet were thin enough to be folded, rolled, or fluffed for a variety of purposes.

As I was packing to come home from the hospital, my nurse started stacking all of my pillows on my cart. She told me they were disposable and would be thrown away if I left them in my room, so I might as well take them.

I was so glad I did because I then kept several on my bed upstairs, several in my recliner chair in the family room downstairs, and even in my car to use with my seat belt. Since I distributed them everywhere I needed them, I didn't have to carry them from place to place. They were a huge factor in helping me settle into more comfortable positions.

Before leaving the hospital, ask if your pillows are going to be sanitized and reused or if they are going to be thrown out. If they will be discarded, by all means take them home with you.

Memory Loss

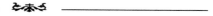

TIP: **This may be the only time in your life when you will have a legitimate excuse for not being able to remember names, important information, or other details. It is short term memory that is affected.**

One thing that can sometimes follow a lengthy surgery is having a slow memory. I simply could not remember people's names, times I took medications, where I put things, or who I had talked to on the phone. This was especially true if I had to respond quickly. It just wasn't there; I only had a big, blank void. A little time and several hints occasionally helped. Otherwise, it just took time.

I was convinced I was experiencing the early stages of permanent memory loss, but was told this is not uncommon. It could be due to the residual effects from the anesthesia, medication or even the experience of dealing with breast cancer. It can affect some people more than others. It was a relief knowing I had a legitimate excuse for not remembering things—even if it was only temporary.

Jim had a much more difficult time understanding what I was experiencing than I did. If he asked me who brought us dinner, I might say, "the blonde from church." I knew exactly who she was, what she did, and how many children she had, but I simply could not remember her name. I even knew who her husband was, but of course, I couldn't remember his name either. Jim and I would play the guessing game and then I would get so excited when he would come up with the right name!

After about eight weeks, my memory slowly started returning or at least it was close to being back to where it was prior to surgery—not perfect, but improved. I don't know how long I'll be able to use this as an excuse, but I'll use it as long as I can.

Sneezing, Coughing, Laughing

──────────────── ❧☀❧ ────────────────

TIP: **Sneezing after abdominal surgery is as much fun as diving into a pool without water. Avoid it any way you can!**

Trust me ... I *did not* want to sneeze for a month or two after having a TRAM. If my nose started to tingle, I immediately pinched my nostrils together in an effort to stop the oncoming sneeze.

If this didn't work, I would literally drop everything from both hands, bend forward, and hold onto my abdomen. This was not the time for me to have a dainty "ah-choo," but instead I would let it go full force. Because I was curled up in a ball with my head down, I was not worried about spreading germs. It also helped if I had time to grab a pillow and hold it across my abdomen before bending forward.

Coughing and laughing are definitely not much better, but the above method works there, too. The good news is that this improves with time.

Speed Bumps

──────────────── ❧☀❧ ────────────────

TIP: **WARNING! The combination of a speed bump, a seat belt, and a TRAM are to be handled with extreme caution (Refer to the previous tip regarding sneezing). Be aware of speed bumps at all times.**

It wasn't long before Jim and I learned a valuable lesson: you must always be on the lookout for the land mines they call speed bumps. I'll never forget going over my first speed bump as we were leaving the hospital parking lot. My first thought was, "This was a real test to see if my paper tape is going to hold my abdominal incision together." At that point, I definitely wished I had insisted on duct tape!

When my daughters or friends would drive me places, this was always the first warning I would give them. I kept my eyes glued to the road, always on the lookout. I would yell way in advance for the driver to slow down almost to a complete stop and then slowly roll over the bumps. I would take my free hand and stretch my seat belt out as far as it would go and hold my other hand on my stomach. I also learned that the dips at driveway entrances could be just as painful as speed bumps.

Mini Pads and Nursing Pads

———————————— 之柰彡 ————————————

TIP: **There are multiple and creative uses for mini pads and nursing pads. Don't be afraid (or embarrassed) to use them.**

I panicked early one morning about ten days after surgery. When I took my nightshirt off to get into the shower, I noticed several dark spots at the level of my mastectomy. Thank goodness I already had a follow-up appointment with my surgeon the following day. I decided I would wait and mention it to him then.

When I found several more spots on my blouse later in the day, I decided I should go ahead and call him just in case there was a problem. I talked with a nurse who said it was not unusual and they would definitely check it when I came in the next day. She said to cover it with a small gauze pad to protect my clothes.

The next day when I showed it to my surgeon, he asked if I had any mini pads at home. Although I thought this was strange, I remembered I did still have several. He suggested I tape one over the area that was draining for several days until it cleared up. This was a first—using a mini pad over my new breast! Nursing pads will also work, but it had been 30 years since I had any of those in my house!

On the Road Again

꿎本꿏

TIP: **Ask your surgeon how long you must wait before you are allowed to drive.**

At my two-week post-op appointment, my doctor gave me the okay to drive. Although I was excited, I was also nervous, especially since my abdomen was still tight and my chest was sore when I used my arms.

Somewhat nervous, I waited until after dinner that night when I knew there would not be much traffic. I picked up my keys and casually told Jim I was going for a test drive in the neighborhood. Taking my time, I slowly drove over the dip at the end of our driveway. As my confidence increased, I decided to venture onto back roads where there weren't many cars. Before I realized it, I was cruising around the downtown area of Cumming, near my home.

It was an absolutely beautiful summer evening—warm, but not hot. Now totally confident, I rolled down all of the windows, opened the sunroof, and turned the volume on the radio a little louder than usual. Now that I think about it, it was *much* louder than usual. I hesitated as I approached the entrance ramp. After hesitating only briefly, I turned and increased my speed as I entered the highway. My short hair was blowing in the breeze. I had forgotten how much fun it was to drive. It felt so good to be independent again!

I called Jim so he wouldn't worry about why my drive "in the neighborhood" was taking so long. About 45 minutes later, I turned into the driveway only to find he had closed the garage door! No way did I want to call him on my cell phone and ask for help!

I sat there staring up at the remote button, and realized there was no way I could raise my arm high enough to reach it. Looking around the car, I found a pen. It was just barely long enough to make contact with the button and raise the garage door.

Afterwards, Jim made the comment, "You are just like a teenager who has gotten her driver's license for the first time!" You bet I was and I loved every minute of that night's drive.

Toupee Tape

TIP: Toupee tape is great for keeping necklines closed or close against your skin so no one gets an unexpected sneak peek of your surgery sites.

This is a tip I learned from my sister, Linda, long before I needed it after surgery. I have used toupee tape to keep bra straps from slipping off my shoulder, to mend a loose hem, to keep sling-back shoes from slipping on my heels, etc. The list is endless.

Two months after surgery I attended a formal event at a conference in New York. The dress I wanted to wear had a large ruffle around the neck that plunged to a low V in the front. It stayed in place if I held my shoulders back and didn't move. But standing still was going to be impossible since the event included a seated dinner. I also knew I would be meeting new people as well as seeing friends I had not seen since before my surgery. I really didn't want to wear a high-necked dress as if I was hiding something. I wanted to look my best so they could see how great I was doing.

All of a sudden, I remembered my toupee tape! I simply taped the open, low-cut neckline directly to my skin. I felt fabulous and especially enjoyed the positive comments I received when everyone realized I was only eight weeks post-op from having a bilateral mastectomy. I didn't realize removing the tape would be as hard as it was, but it sure was worth it.

I always buy a box of generic brand strips at a beauty supply store. Since they are wider than I need, I cut them in half lengthwise and have twice as many.

Rx Bras

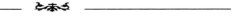

TIP: **Even after having reconstruction following a mastectomy, special bras are available and fitted by nurses trained in this service. Check with your insurance company to see if they cover this expense. Mine paid for two bras the first year and will pay for one per year after that.**

I never thought I would get a prescription for a bra! On one of my follow-up office visits to my plastic surgeon, I asked when I would be able to start wearing a bra again and if there were any limitations. I was surprised when he wrote out a prescription and told me to take it to the Women's Center at the hospital where they would fit me with a bra.

There was really no need for me to rush, but at age 60 I had never gone braless and wasn't used to it. I was anxious and went way too soon after surgery. After I wore it back home, I realized it was not as comfortable as going braless. It looked exactly like a sports bra, but with a front closure.

For the time being, I went back to wearing my loose fitting camisoles that were oh so comfortable. That was another time I wish I'd had more patience and waited until I had healed a little more. In retrospect, I really didn't need one of the special bras after all.

Mrs. Doubtfire

───────────────── ⚜ ─────────────────

TIP: **There is danger in having larger breasts, especially when you're not used to having them and they don't have any feeling. Be aware of any potential hazards.**

At first it was hard for me to remember I didn't have any feeling in my breasts. Plus, I was not used to them being slightly larger than my natural breasts had been.

One day when I was heating something on my gas stove, I laughed out loud at the thought of Mrs. Doubtfire and her accident in the kitchen when her "stuffing" caught on fire. I can still imagine how easily this could have happened if I had leaned too far over one of my gas burners. I probably wouldn't notice until my eyelashes were singed!

Then again, I knew this wouldn't happen since I am not known for cooking very often. My philosophy is that just because I am a woman, that doesn't mean I know how to, enjoy, or want to cook. I retired from cooking when our youngest child went to college. Rarely, if ever, am I in front of my stove!

Some of the feeling has gradually returned to my breasts and my abdomen. But I still don't plan on standing in front of any burners.

Physical Therapy

───────────────── ⚜ ─────────────────

TIP: **Be aware that there are physical therapists trained in treating post-mastectomy patients.**

At a booth at the Expo for the Atlanta 2-Day Walk for Breast Cancer training event, I met a physical therapist who specialized in working with post-mastectomy patients. She worked at a facility called Turning Point that offers a variety of programs for breast cancer survivors. My breast surgeon wrote a prescription for me to see if they could work out a lingering "hot spot" I had on the underside of one of my arms.

At three months post-op, I had full mobility in both of my arms and shoulders. But whenever someone touched the back part of my left upper arm, I would jump and feel like I was being stung by a bee. Jim was the person this happened to the most, and he could not understand why the back of my arm was so sensitive when all of my surgery had been on the front of my body.

The physical therapist evaluated my condition and showed me stretches and exercises I could easily do at home. Within a month, my "hot spot" was gone.

Good Days and Great Days

TIP: Go with the flow and take each day as it comes. If you don't happen to be having a spectacular day, remember these words: "This too shall pass."

For the most part, I felt pretty good considering the surgery I had just experienced. There were some post-operative days I felt really great and there were some when I just wanted to sit and not do a thing. If I didn't have much energy, I would rationalize by saying it was my body's way of telling me to slow down and take the time to heal.

It didn't take long for me to realize that whenever I pushed myself too much on one day, I would know I needed to plan on resting more the following day. It was interesting how it almost fell into an "every other day" pattern. I didn't have any regrets about being active on my "feel good" days because I knew I would just plan on taking it easy the following day.

Follow-Up Surgery

Tip: **Take advantage of this opportunity to select your breast size. The options in breast reconstruction are amazing. If you had large breasts prior to your mastectomy, you can opt for a breast reduction during the reconstruction. If you want to keep your pre-surgery size, then replacements can be exactly the same size. And if you had small breasts all of your life and want to fulfill a dream of finally having cleavage, you can opt for an enlargement – another example of the pink lemonade approach!**

I had more issues dealing with the reconstructive segment of surgery than I did with having the mastectomy. In my mind, I felt I should have just been thrilled that my cancer had been removed and not be concerned with what size my breasts would be after the reconstruction.

My plastic surgeon told me that after what I had experienced having a mastectomy, I should be 100% pleased with the final results. This was my opportunity to have whatever size I wanted, within reason. I was so nervous that if I said I wanted to be larger, I would end up too top-heavy for my frame. If I said I wanted to be small, I was afraid I would end up being smaller than I was prior to surgery, although I'm not sure that was possible.

During my first visit with him, I remember he mentioned that although I didn't have much stomach fat, he still suggested the TRAM because I had excess skin from carrying three large babies. My smallest was seven pounds, 13 ounces and my largest was nine pounds, five ounces and we all know skin only shrinks so much. Using my own tissues would result in having soft, natural breasts. If after surgery, I was smaller than I wanted to be, he could easily put in small artificial implants. We would do this about four months after the mastectomy and at the same time as the nipple reconstruction.

After much deliberation, this is what I decided to do. The surgery did require having tubes again, but only two this time. Because of my work (I had speaking engagements on the calendar), I waited until mid-November, which was five months post-op.

I am definitely pleased with my decision. If at 90 I decide I'm too "perky," I can always have the artificial implants removed and still have breasts.

CHAPTER 7

Additional Treatments

At about six weeks post-op, my breast surgeon referred me to an oncologist for evaluation and follow-up. At first, I was surprised that I would have an oncologist because I didn't have a lumpectomy and radiation and the post-surgery pathology report revealed no other cancer present in either of my breasts or in any of my lymph nodes.

However, I felt confident knowing that many of my "breast friends" also went to this same oncologist. After reviewing all of my records and taking into consideration that my cancer was found and treated while it was still small (0.7 centimeters) and was not in my lymph nodes, my oncologist said I was not a candidate for chemotherapy. She started me on Femara, which is a drug treatment for postmenopausal women who have had early stage breast cancer. Its purpose is to reduce the risk of cancer returning.

Part of me was relieved not to have chemo and another part was disappointed because I had made a commitment early on that I would treat my cancer as aggressively as possible. I thought at the very least I might have at least one or two doses of chemo.

Although I didn't have chemo myself, several of my "breast friends" suggested I include a section with tips for women who will be having it. I appreciated their offer to share their thoughts. Remember, these are their experiences. The bottom line is for you to ask questions and discuss the details of your treatment with your oncologist.

Radiation

―――――――――――――― と本ら ――――――――――――――

Make conserving your energy and moisturizing your skin a high priority.

I was surprised that the time it took to receive each radiation treatment was similar to the time it took to have an x-ray or a mammogram. The time it took to undress and get into position was far longer than the time it took to actually receive the radiation.

For the entire time that I received treatments, I literally had no energy and was exhausted. It became my mission to conserve my energy.

Treatments reminded me of getting sunburned. To help keep my skin moist, a nurse suggested I rub vitamin E oil on the radiation site immediately after each treatment, after bathing, and before going to bed. This proved to be a tremendous help.

Marcia Steele

Chemotherapy

―――――――――――――― と本ら ――――――――――――――

TIP: **Be aware that your oncology team cares about you and wants to do their best to help you through this experience. When you go to the chemo lab, look for other patients who have positive attitudes. Use this opportunity to make new friends.**

I didn't know what to expect when I first entered the chemo lab, but I embraced it. My motto was "Chemo is my friend" – and it has been!

The thought of chemo can be a little frightening, to say the very least, but I found it peaceful and comforting. I am so grateful that the doctor had a high standard of care for my cancer. Yes, there are side effects, but I received excellent care and was monitored carefully. If I had any discomfort, the doctor had a solution and made every effort to keep me comfortable and keep my energy levels up.

I met new friends each time I went to the chemo lab. We shared our stories with each other. I looked forward to seeing these dear friends each time I went for treatments.

For me, the chemo lab was a cheerful place. The nurses and staff were loving, committed, and caring professionals who made me feel welcome. They did their best to make me comfortable while I was in their care.

Debbie Beall

Fatigue, Taste, Nails

TIP: Ask doctors, nurses, and other chemotherapy patients for tips they can share to combat side effects.

When my pathology report revealed breast cancer was in my lymph nodes, I was scared. I approached it as a bump in the road of life and I took it one day at a time. As it turned out, it wasn't too bad.

All of the horrible things I had heard about chemo came rushing in—fatigue, nausea, loss of taste ... and then I heard one of the drugs I would be taking may damage my fingernails. The fatigue and loss of taste were the worst. I ate what I could taste, which was mostly spicy Mexican foods and sweets. Of course, instead of losing weight while on chemo, I gained 15 pounds!

To combat the fatigue, they suggested exercise, which probably would have helped limit the weight gain. I was really whipped and gave in to daily naps. To me that was *my* time. Besides, I wasn't sleeping well anyway at night, so I slept when I could.

I did have some issues with my fingernails splitting and being soft. I learned in a Chemoflage class that if I kept my nails in a cup of ice while receiving treatment, it would help them stay healthy. I used a cold pack on my toenails because it did affect both.

Debbie Tucker

Passing the Time

──────────────── ༄༅ ────────────────

TIP: **Find ways to keep yourself occupied while you're in the chemotherapy lab.**

──────────────────────────────────

Plan ahead for the time you will be spending in the chemo lab. Some of the time, I spent exercising my brain by working Sudoku puzzles, and other times I just rested.

I laughed when I read that Martha also solved Sudoku puzzles while sitting in waiting rooms in doctors' offices, labs, admissions, and even before surgery, because I did exactly the same thing, especially during the time I spent in the chemo lab. I knew working those puzzles would help my mind, and besides, I enjoyed the challenge. It wasn't long before I had mastered the beginner series and then the medium. Now I have even become quite an expert with the advanced puzzles. It has been a great way to pass the time and still feel productive.

Peggy

Hair Loss and Wigs

──────────────── ༄༅ ────────────────

TIP: **Remember that hair is just hair; it's not what makes you who you are.**

──────────────────────────────────

I would have never cut my hair short, but chemo helped me see that hair is just hair. It is what is underneath your hair that makes you who you are.

The issue with losing hair is a big deal, especially for women. Most women think that if you are having a bad hair day, then your day will not be perfect. Oh how *unimportant* I realized my hair was!

Before chemo, I had a full head of thick, long hair. Because I didn't think I could handle the emotion of waking up and finding it all on my pillow or falling off in my hands in the shower, I chose to shave it off before it fell out. For me, this was the best choice.

My niece met me at the store where I picked out my wigs. I bought one that day so I could wear it as soon as they buzzed my head. It was great. I thought I would just break down and cry, but I didn't. They were so helpful and caring. Of course we then went to a Mexican restaurant and had chips, salsa, and margaritas!

As a side note, I went a little overboard with the purchase of wigs. I bought three—a short one I named Sassy, a medium-length one named Sophie, and a long one I named Sexy. When my friends called, they would each ask, "Who are you today—Sassy, Sophie, or Sexy?" The wigs were all my natural hair color, and I admit I wore Sophie more than I did the others. Those wigs were definitely an impulse buy, but they did help me cope.

My hair started growing back even during chemo. But after my last chemo treatment, I lost hair again. A few weeks after that it began to grow and thicken. It has now come back thicker and curlier than it has ever been. The bright side to this is that it is easy to fix and very stylish. I love my new hair!

Debbie Tucker

Human Water Filter

TIP: **Remember to stay hydrated during chemotherapy treatments.**

In addition to the fluids included at the time of your chemo, drink water while you are receiving your treatment. Staying hydrated during and after my chemo treatments helped me pass the toxins out of my body.

Even when I didn't feel like taking a shower each day, I did. I washed thoroughly with a mild soap. This not only opened my pores, but it also made me feel better. Also, I found that something as simple as wearing lipstick and getting dressed rather than staying in pajamas also helped boost my spirits and made me feel so much better.

Marcia Steele

CHAPTER 8

The Future

I used to tell my audiences, "I plan on living to be at least 101." If I hadn't been diagnosed with breast cancer, I now realize I probably wouldn't have even lived to be 71, at least not with the fast pace I was keeping. I was always dealing with far more self-induced stress than I care to confess, and I typically consumed a diet of fast food and anything sweet.

Being diagnosed with cancer was a huge wakeup call for me. I realized my priorities were totally out of line. Before I had cancer, if you had asked me if I thought my health was important, I would have said, "Definitely, yes." I thought it was among my top priorities, yet I ate junk food, candy, and desserts, never had time to exercise, stayed up late at night, and never seemed to get enough sleep.

Through my research and experiences, I have learned what a vital role good nutrition and exercise can play in maintaining good health. I have learned to stress less and pay more attention to the things that matter the most to me. It is all a matter of establishing priorities.

Stress Management

TIP: **Before you allow yourself to be stressed, evaluate the situation. If there is nothing you can do about it, then let it go. If there is something you can do about it, don't procrastinate; just go ahead and do it!**

For years, I felt like a duck that appeared to be just floating on the surface. However, beneath the water, my feet were paddling at 150 miles per hour! Prior to being diagnosed, my stress level had totally maxed out! My plate was not just full, but overflowing! What was so amazing was that I finally realized my stress was all self-induced.

Once I learned through my research what a vital role stress plays in my overall health, I made a personal commitment to eliminate it! I just stopped worrying about what I couldn't control and focused on what I could control.

Traffic no longer bothered me because I either left earlier or listened to my favorite CDs. While waiting for doctor appointments or lab tests, I worked on Sudoku puzzles or just took time to relax and enjoy my surroundings.

Today if I feel anxiety creeping up on me again, I remind myself to take a deep breath and stop wasting my time or energy sweating the small stuff.

Exercise for the Health of It

TIP: **Make a commitment to start and maintain an exercise program, even if it is just walking. Regular exercise increases your stamina and level of energy. Besides speeding your recovery from surgery, it also helps fight heart disease, diabetes and osteoporosis. Make sure to exercise regularly.**

As soon as my daughters learned that my surgeon told me I could physically do anything I wanted, they reissued their challenge for me to compete in a triathlon. This time I accepted without any hesitation!

I registered for the Aflac Iron Girl Sprint Triathlon scheduled for June 28, 2009. This is the same event I had cancelled a year earlier because of having surgery. Several weeks after registering, a friend told me about a First Timers triathlon which was scheduled several weeks earlier on June 6. I also registered for this one thinking it would be great preparation for the Aflac Iron Girl.

Today I am in the best physical condition of my life. The secret to staying healthy and feeling young is exercise. I plan on dancing at all seven of my grandchildren's weddings. I will only be 91 if the youngest (to date) is 30 when she gets married!

Seminars and Education

TIP: Check with your hospital for a list of non-profit agencies that offer educational courses and additional resources.

At the breast cancer orientation meeting I attended at the hospital prior to my surgery, I was given a pamphlet with a two-month calendar showing upcoming events offered by The Wellness Community. This is a non-profit organization affiliated with my hospital. Most hospitals have a connection with a similar organization. The Wellness Community offers such programs as nutrition classes, yoga, Pilates, support groups, luncheons, and educational programs presented by a variety of doctors and specialists. There are additional locations throughout the country. Log onto http://www.theWellnessCommunity.com.

While attending programs and learning more about surviving breast cancer, I developed lasting friendships with so many incredible women. Many of the programs and events are sponsored by It's The Journey, which is supported by funds raised from the Atlanta 2-Day Walk for Breast Cancer and from Susan G. Komen for the Cure. *All* are totally free to cancer survivors!

Nutrition Tips

——————————— ぞ本ら ——————————

TIP: **Eating a healthy, well-balanced diet is the key to good nutrition. It is recommended to eat three servings of fruit and five servings of vegetables every day.**

As I've mentioned before, the fact that I am a woman doesn't mean I know how to cook, want to cook, or enjoy cooking. For 25 years I prepared well-balanced meals for my husband and three children. When our last child left home to attend college, I announced to my family that I was retiring from cooking.

I still don't like to cook, but I can press a button. The nutritionist at The Wellness Community recommended a heavy-duty juicer. I bought one that is so strong it grinds pulp and even the seeds so you don't lose any nutrients (Thanks again, Aflac). The motor is so strong I'm sure you could ski behind it. Juicing is one way for me to have my five servings of veggies a day. My veggie shakes taste so much better when I drink them from a stemmed, crystal water goblet.

From attending the nutrition classes at The Wellness Community, I have learned what constitutes a healthy, well-balanced diet. These classes are offered twice a month throughout the year and offer great tips on which foods are good for us and how to prepare them. The classes are led by a medical nutrition therapist who has been fabulous in sharing her expertise.

Post-Mastectomy Yoga

——————————— ぞ本ら ——————————

TIP: **Yoga classes structured for post-mastectomy and reconstructive surgery are a great resource for gradually stretching your muscles, learning deep breathing exercises and discovering how to relax your mind and body through meditation.**

When I learned that The Wellness Community was offering yoga classes, I thought I would at least go check them out, especially since they were advertised as "stress reduction." This was another one of the free programs offered to cancer survivors.

I was six weeks post-op when I attended my first class. There were five other women there—all yoga veterans and breast cancer survivors for many years. By this time, I was able to stand upright, but my abdomen was still extremely tight. The instructor helped me modify several of the more strenuous exercises. By the time the class was over, I felt my muscles relaxing and gradually becoming looser.

During the last 15 minutes of class she told us to lie down on our mats and relax. Several of the women rested the calves of their legs on the seat of a chair. Not to be left out, I followed suit. We each covered ourselves with the towels we had brought. The instructor dimmed the lights and played a CD with beautiful, relaxing music.

From this peaceful bliss, I was awakened by a loud, guttural, gasping sound. I had woken myself up snoring! I was so embarrassed. After that, I decided never to lie flat on my back again during the meditation part of yoga class.

Support Groups

TIP: **Don't try to do it alone, especially when there are so many women who have traveled this road before you and have experienced what you are feeling. Also, as survivors, we can help those following behind us.**

At about six weeks post-op, I attended my first support group sponsored by The Wellness Community. I had no idea what to expect. I was hesitant at first, thinking it may be sad or depressing, but I decided I would attend at least one meeting. I was pleasantly surprised to find it quite the opposite.

I met the most amazing group of women. Most of them were long-time survivors who had treatment years ago but still enjoyed getting together once every month. I felt like the new kid on the block and I appreciated their warmth and kindness as they welcomed me into their group.

I was both intrigued and reassured as they shared brief snippets of their experiences. What I loved the best was how we mostly laughed and had fun.

Check with your surgeon, hospital, or with other breast cancer survivors for information on support groups in your area.

Think Positive

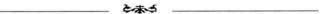

TIP: **Focus your thoughts on all the good things that result from being a breast cancer survivor.**

I am a firm believer that situations improve when we focus on the positive. This works with all aspects of life, not just having breast cancer. Here are several positives from my list:

- Didn't have to vacuum or clean the house for about three months after surgery
- Didn't have to cook because meals were provided for several weeks
- Was given the opportunity to rethink and refocus my life and my future
- Learned more about breast cancer
- Met some of the most incredible people, especially women
- Learned about nutrition and eating healthy
- Exercised more, which helped my overall health
- Now have new breasts that are larger than my original ones

- Have breasts that will still look perky when I'm 90 (or older)
- Eliminated belly flab left over from pregnancies with three big babies
- Gained the opportunity to help other women in similar situations
- Walked 30 miles in the Atlanta 2-Day Walk for Breast Cancer
- Raised almost $4,000 as a participant in the Atlanta 2-Day Walk for Breast Cancer
- Wrote a book
- Gained the opportunity to empower women
- Invited to bowl with several of the Atlanta Falcon football players
- Asked to speak at the closing ceremony for the Atlanta 2-Day Walk for Breast Cancer
- Asked to emcee and participate at the DeKalb Adams Relay for Life sponsored by the American Cancer Society
- Facilitated a panel of distinguished doctors and specialists at Piedmont Hospital on the latest breast cancer facts

Accept the Love

TIP: **Put yourself in a position to receive the love from those who feel close to you.**

Finally being able to drive again gave me back my freedom. I am sure I looked ridiculous with one pillow across my lap, another one straight up protecting my chest, and the seatbelt stretched to the max.

I had only been driving again for three days when I decided I would attend the monthly meeting of my local chapter of the National Speakers Association. Although a fellow member who lived nearby offered to drive me, I insisted on driving myself. I told him that if I felt tired, I would be able to leave early. If I felt okay, I could stay for the full day!

Although it was an hour's drive to get there, I really wanted to go. I had served as president of the chapter the previous year and I was anxious to see my good friends and colleagues again.

I woke up earlier than usual (I guess I was excited) and had time to shower, dress, and arrive in time for the board meeting prior to the main session. It was such a boost to see the surprised expressions on everyone's faces. No one expected me to be there so soon after surgery.

During our meetings we have an exercise called "pass the microphone" when each person has about ten seconds to stand up and give their name and area of expertise. For as long as I live, I will never forget what happened when it was my turn. I took the microphone and slowly pushed back my chair. I strained to stand as tall I could. I was only able to say my name before being interrupted by applause and a standing ovation from everyone in the room.

Words cannot describe my shock and surprise at their thoughtfulness. The love and support I felt at that moment from my colleagues is one that I will cherish and remember forever.

New Opportunities

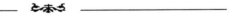

TIP: **Stretch yourself, both mentally and physically, and do something you have never done before.**

When I was out walking shortly after my surgery, I saw two of my neighbors, Doug and Becky. They told me told me about the Atlanta 2-Day Walk for Breast Cancer. During my six-week follow-up visit, I asked my surgeon if he thought I would be able to walk 30 miles just three and a half months after my surgery. I thought he would say no and let me off the hook.

He said if I felt like it, I should go for it. I had my doubts, because I had never walked more than three miles at any time in my life and that was just prior to surgery when I had been training for the sprint triathlon. Becky offered to walk with me to help me get in shape. On mornings when my bed was warm and comfortable, I knew she was waiting for me. She was a tremendous support in being an accountability partner.

At only seven-and-a-half weeks post-op, I registered as a participant and attended my first training walk. I had the option of walking either six miles or 12 miles. Mind you, my abdomen was still tight from the abdominal surgery and I had only recently worked my way back to walking three miles in my neighborhood. I was thinking it would be a miracle if I could manage to finish the six-mile course!

During the warm-up, I met another recent breast cancer survivor who had the same plastic surgeon I had. Her surgery had been about two months before mine. When we reached the fork where we had to decide on taking the six-mile or the 12-mile course, she talked me into going with her on the longer route. We knew if we couldn't make it, we could sit on the curb and one of the staff would drive by and pick us up.

We had so much fun talking, laughing, and sharing our experiences that the time and the miles passed quickly. When we realized we had already walked 11 miles and only had a mile to go, we were both surprised and thrilled! After we finished you would have thought we had just finished the Boston Marathon! I knew then I would not have a problem walking thirty miles two months later in the Atlanta 2-Day Walk for Breast Cancer.

Even with late registration, I was able to raise almost $4,000! My two daughters walked with me and we had an incredible experience. Another highlight was being asked to speak during the closing ceremonies. That was another experience I will always remember!

You can go to the following website to see pictures from the event and learn more about this incredible organization: http://www.itsthe-journey. org.

Have Fun (My Madonna Moment)
————————— 🐛🎋🐟 —————————

TIP: Being able to laugh at yourself makes you feel better and helps ease concerns expressed by your family, friends, and colleagues.

I mentioned earlier about my trip to New York and dressing for the formal dinner. Here is something I did at the same conference just to have fun.

The event was the National Speakers Association (NSA) annual convention. The theme throughout the year had been "NSA Rocks." All year long the events were related in some way to rock bands, rock stars, concerts, tours, etc. For the opening ceremony, they instructed all attendees to come dressed like rock stars. This would have really been cool if at least three-fourths of the attendees, or even half, had dressed as they were told. As it turned out, only 50 of 1,900 people followed the instructions, which made those of us who did dress up rather conspicuous.

Because the convention was only two months after my surgery, I didn't decide until the last minute to attend. I called my niece, Wendy, who is a costume guru, for suggestions. She came up with the wildest idea but was not totally sure I had the nerve to do it. I not only surprised her, but everyone at the conference, once they figured out it was me in the Madonna costume—cones and all!

I was able to find a blonde wig, black lace fingerless gloves and ankle socks, silver chain necklaces, a wide silver-sequined belt, thirty bangle bracelets on each arm, a short black top, knee-length tights, black high heels, pale makeup, and a black mole beneath my right nostril. I made the cones from the cardboard filters used to pour oil into your car. I stapled six of them together for each side to keep them stiff, colored them with black magic marker, cut out the cups from a black bra, and shoved them through the openings. Although they only stuck out about six inches, they were deadly! I still can't believe I did this, although I have the pictures to remind me.

Because people didn't know how I was dealing with having a mastectomy and breast cancer or what they should say to me, I wanted my friends to know I was not just okay, but doing great and able to laugh about it all!

Cut Yourself Some Slack

TIP: **Don't try to be an invincible, indestructible superstar. Take advantage of this time because you will never have this opportunity again.**

This tip is also for my benefit. There were times throughout the first several months of my recovery when I thought I could do anything I wanted to do and then became discouraged because I got so tired.

I'll never forget seeing my oncologist for the first time and sharing how frustrated I was when there was something I wanted to do but did not have the energy. She paused, leaned toward me, looked directly into my eyes and said, "Lighten up and cut yourself some slack. If ever in your lifetime you have a right to relax and slow down, *now* is the time."

I realized *I* was the one person who was pushing me; no one else was. This was probably the only time when no one expected me to do anything other than rest and recuperate. Even today, when I begin to feel overloaded I remember her words, lighten my load, and give myself permission to slow down.

Breast Friends

TIP: **The new friends you will meet will be some of the greatest, most incredible friends you will ever have.**

The women I have met throughout this journey are like none other. I think our biggest link is that we have a new outlook on living. We share a deep camaraderie that words simply cannot describe.

As I mentioned earlier, Debbie and I became close "breast friends" after the breast cancer orientation program we attended at the hospital prior to our surgery.

Several weeks later, Debbie met another new friend at one of her chemo treatments and invited her to join us for lunch. Would you believe her name is also Debbie? Now Debbie, Debbie and I meet regularly for a nutritious lunch, usually at Sweet Tomatoes. We are like the three musketeers.

Because our situations were so similar, we would frequently compare our progress. We asked each other questions we couldn't ask anyone else and knew we would get honest answers.

Each time we get together, I know people are wondering who we are and why we are laughing so hard. If they only knew! I feel blessed to have these two very, very special friends.

Share the Love

TIP: **You never know what kind of day another survivor is having or how she is feeling. Look her in the eye, tell her how wonderful she is, and give her a gentle hug.**

At the beginning of my journey, I wasn't really sure what type of support I wanted or needed, much less what other survivors wanted or needed. I quickly realized that everyone enjoys feeling loved and feeling special.

Being noticed in a caring way provides a huge boost. I appreciated the kind words, but most of all, I loved the hugs. I always laughed inside when a non-breast cancer survivor approached me. I could tell they wanted to hug, but at the same time were afraid to get too close to me. Because other people were often more uptight than I was, I thought about wearing a button that said, "Hugs welcome!" Other survivors will always give you a great big bear hug and never give it a second thought.

Teach Others

かみ

TIP: **One of the best lessons shared is one that is learned from experience.**

Although I never had the good fortune to meet Cavett Robert, the founder of the National Speakers Association, I have heard many great things about him. He believed in learning by "OPE"—Other People's Experiences. We can learn so much from the mistakes, experiences, and successes of others. Living with cancer is no exception.

When I was diagnosed, I had the option of keeping the diagnosis private or shouting it from the rooftops. I chose the latter, in hopes that my journey would make the road easier for those who followed. My wish is for people to learn from my experience so their journey will be much smoother.

Hardly a week goes by that someone doesn't call to tell me a friend of theirs has just been diagnosed with breast cancer. They want to know if it is okay to give their friend my name and number, and if I would mind talking with them.

This is one of the reasons I decided to write this book. I felt there was a need to provide answers to questions people might have or not even know to ask, as well as give positive feedback from my experience. I thoroughly enjoy talking with anyone who has questions or just wants to talk.

Sisterhood

TIP: Once a woman has been diagnosed with breast cancer, she enters a place where camaraderie is taken to a level higher than she can ever imagine. It is a sisterhood made up of truly unique women.

Several months after my mastectomy, I went shopping. All summer I had been wearing baggy clothes. Now I was ready to get back into style. I had speaking engagements in several weeks and I wanted something new to wear.

I went to my favorite store and I started pulling clothes off of the racks. I liked everything I saw. It didn't take long before my arms were loaded. The sweetest sales lady came over and offered to take the clothes and reserve a dressing room for me. I blurted out, "You better save two because I'm a recent breast cancer survivor and I see so many things I want to try on."

You would have thought I had announced this over the loud speaker! Three different women who overheard my comment came up to me out of nowhere, offered congratulations, and said they were survivors too. Once total strangers, we now had an instant friendship as they welcomed me into their "sisterhood."

I wear my pink bracelet or pink ribbon pin just about everywhere I go. Frequently, women come up to me and ask how long I've been a survivor or, at the very least, give me the sweetest smile knowing that we share so much in common.

Dream List

TIP: Wherever you place your focus is what manifests in your life. Take the time to think seriously about what you would like to do in your lifetime. Think big and be willing to face your fears and stretch your comfort zone. Start making a list, put it where you will see it often, and continuously add new ideas.

It wasn't until several years ago that I started making my dream lists. I like taking it a step further by cutting out pictures and gluing them onto a large poster board in my office where I see it every day.

Some of the items on my dream list include:

- A guest appearance on *Oprah* to inform more women about early breast cancer detection
- Walk yearly in the Atlanta 2-Day Walk for Breast Cancer
- Own a cottage in the mountains of north Georgia
- Spend a week at the beach with all of our children and grandchildren
- Walk yearly in the Susan G. Komen 3-Day Walk for Breast Cancer
- Sponsor comedy events for breast cancer survivors
- Buy a road bike and all the equipment I'll need to compete in triathlons (done)
- Have a pool membership and swim at least twice weekly (done)
- Join a Masters swim team
- Finish a triathlon and become a Triathlete (done)
- Finish a marathon
- Go on a foreign mission trip with my church

- Start a foundation to raise funds to help breast cancer survivors
- Own a condo at the beach in Seagrove, Florida
- Go on an African safari (photographic)
- Go white water rafting
- Bike across the state (or the country?)
- Take all of our children and grandchildren on a Disney Cruise
- Publish five additional books

For immediate goals I want to achieve in the current year, I type each of my top three on separate pages in a large font. Then I list all of the reasons why I want to achieve them along with the benefits. For each goal, I print three duplicate pages, take them to Office Max, and have each of the sheets laminated. Then I place them on my desk, tape them to the wall in front of my treadmill or on my bathroom mirror, put them in my sports bag, and even put them in my car.

Subtle Reminders

────────────────── と本ざ ──────────────────

TIP: **A pinch, a pull, a person, or a place can trigger a gentle reminder of your journey.**

I am sure there will come a time when the strange and unique tingles, aches, and weird feelings I have will vanish, but until then I consider them gentle reminders of my experience and how thrilled I am to be alive. I am reminded of my journey every morning when I take the Femara medication prescribed by my oncologist. It decreases the chances of my cancer returning somewhere else in my body. Ironically, this tiny little pill is exactly the same size my cancer was.

There are some things I will always remember. Every time I park in front of T.J. Maxx, I remember the exact spot where I parked the day my internist called telling me I needed a repeat chest x-ray. I'll never put my cell phone on the security belt at an airport without remembering the call I received in Seattle telling me the ultrasound indicated I needed to see a breast surgeon.

Each time I eat at Sweet Tomatoes, I think of how much fun my "breast friends" and I have when we get together for lunch. When I drive down Roswell Road, I remember the day I walked 12 miles for the very first time while training for the Atlanta 2-Day Walk for Breast Cancer.

I cherish the memories of each of these special events because they are not just reminders of my past, but encouragement for my future.

Number One Priority

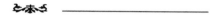

TIP: **Give yourself the gift of extreme self-care and you will not only increase your value to yourself, but also to others.**

Surviving breast cancer has helped me realize the value in taking care of *my* needs first—*100% totally guilt free!* I learned that as much as I love my family, enjoy my friends, and have the desire to help others, I need to first honor myself. Being a breast cancer survivor has given me an opportunity to reevaluate my priorities on how I spend my time, where I go, what I do, and how I live my life.

Previously, I fell into the same category as most women—a natural nurturer. I often felt I should take care of everyone else's needs before my own. On top of that, I had become a workaholic. Over the years, I would feel like a leftover by the end of the day. It would be late in the evening when I would finally crawl into bed for several hours of much-needed sleep before starting the fast pace all over again the following day.

By always saying "yes" and accepting added responsibility rather than speaking up and saying "no," I was training people that it was all right to depend on me for *anything*. I started practicing saying "no" so it flowed easily whenever I needed to say it. Also, I rehearsed a mental list of responses such as, "Thank you so much for asking, but I am not able to help at this time." After making my declaration, I would not say another word. This helped me become more selective in doing what "I wanted" to do, not just what "someone else asked" me to do.

I have also learned to redirect some of my control issues and lighten up on being a perfectionist. I focus more on what I do best and have learned to put my trust in the expertise of others. I don't sweat the small stuff. Jim has always been helpful, but I depend on him more now, especially once I realized he enjoys helping. It is one way he has been able to deal with me being a breast cancer survivor. He doesn't always do things exactly the way I would do them, but I've learned it is okay.

Just the other night we had a group of friends over and Jim offered to handle all of the food for me. He went to the store and bought great hors d'oeuvres and an absolutely fabulous specialty cake. He did an excellent job preparing and displaying the spread, including making the coffee and icing the beverages. We were standing around in the kitchen talking and eating our dessert when I suddenly noticed we were all using Christmas napkins. This would have been fine had it been December, but it was April! There was a day when this would have really bothered me. I just smiled and realized how lucky I am to have someone who enjoys helping me.

I take longer showers and I enjoy listening to music, going to yoga classes, taking long walks, going on bike rides, and spending more time with my family and friends. I enjoy our grandchildren and love watching them grow and develop right in front of my eyes.

I thoroughly enjoy who I am and what I am doing.

Thriving

An Epilogue

It has been a year since I discovered my lump *and* myself. Experiencing an illness like cancer helped me see who I really am from a different perspective, helped me evaluate my priorities, and gave clarity to my existence.

Like so many people, I thought I was living a fulfilling life, but I now realize how frequently I was just going through the motions, never really taking advantage of the opportunities around me or the skills I possess. My experiences with breast cancer have opened my eyes and given me a better understanding of my purpose in life.

I feel blessed to speak to audiences and share stories about how to invest in themselves -- physically, mentally, and spiritually. I have found most people are just too busy to stop and take the time to think about how they want to live their lives, much less make specific plans or reach for bigger goals. Instead, they just let things happen and worry about making changes only when it is necessary.

Some people say things happen for a reason; some call it fate, while others call it a blessing. For me, my breast cancer diagnosis was a wake-up call. I never dreamed I would ever have breast cancer, but then again no woman does.

Then when the diagnosis was confirmed, I almost felt like I was in a transparent state. Although I threw myself into researching cancer and treatments, this gave me an opportunity to adjust to my new identity—"breast cancer survivor."

Once options were evaluated, treatment decided, and my surgery behind me, I felt like I had been given a new lease on life, a new beginning, a fresh start. There were so many things I once took for granted or just accepted; now whatever I do, I do it with focus and intention. Without these two strengths, I would never have been able to walk 12 miles at only seven-and-a-half weeks post-op or walk 30 miles at three-and-a-half months post-op. And, I *never* would have been able to complete an Aflac Iron Girl Triathlon. I loved proving not just to myself, but to others what I am capable of doing. And I know I haven't even come close to doing so many other once-perceived outrageous achievements.

I am on a mission to squeeze every ounce of living out of every one of my days. There are times I feel so good and have so much energy that I feel like laughing so loud the entire world will hear, but then I'm afraid I'll be arrested for disturbing the peace or someone will think I have lost my mind. All I know is that I want to exhaust all of my opportunities by the time my final day comes.

I joined Hearthstone Lodge which is a swim and fitness facility for seniors that is less than a ten-minute drive from my home (There *are* bonuses for being in the 50-plus age group). The lifeguard helped me improve my stroke and my breathing. I am now able to swim over 1200 meters during practice and am confident this will increase over time.

When I was a little girl, I had a hand-me-down sky blue and white bike. At 61, I am proud to say, "I finally have my very first brand *new* bike." After looking for over a month, I bought a great-looking silver Diamondback road bike. I'm sure it is fast, but for right now, I'm not pushing it past 30 mph. I wish you could see me ride. I look really sharp, especially with my matching silver helmet with pale pink flowers. I learned how and when to shift gears to make it up steep hills. The biggest adjustment was learning how to use the hand brakes. Initially, my brain wanted to pedal backwards like I did some 50 years ago. I even bought a one-piece tri suit, silver and white with several pink lines. I like to think of them as racing stripes.

The most amazing thing happened when I started my training for the triathlon. After adding swimming and biking to my walking, the lingering tightness in my abdomen all but disappeared and my muscles became stronger.

I have passed the one-year anniversary of my mastectomy and celebrated by becoming a triathlete. Because I am a breast cancer survivor, Aflac supported me by paying my registration fee for the Aflac Iron Girl Sprint Triathlon. As part of my training, I competed in a triathlon for first timers in June, 2009. I was not out to set any records, but just to finish the course and enjoy the day, the camaraderie, and the experience. Now my goal is to improve my time with each future triathlon. Before having cancer, I never would have dreamed of doing this!

I admit it is physically hard work training for a triathlon, but completing one is all mental. It is training your mind to convince your body that it can do more than it thinks it can do. This was the same philosophy I used during my recovery.

To celebrate my 50th birthday, Lauren took me skydiving. When I was 60, I had a bilateral mastectomy and abdominal free TRAM. At 61, I competed in my first triathlon. Liz and Lauren haven't decided how we will celebrate my 70th, 80th, 90th, or 100th birthdays, but I can assure you each one will be exciting! If you have a challenge or suggestion you would like us to consider, please send me an email at Martha@MarthaLanier.com. None of us know how long we are going to live; I just want to be prepared should I live to be 101 (or older).

For me, surviving cancer is not necessarily about living a long life, but enjoying the life I am living. It is about living each day with a purpose and with meaning.

Over the past year, I have learned more about life and living from other breast cancer survivors than I could have ever imagined. They are some of the toughest fighters on the face of the earth and demonstrate character and courage. You will not find anyone with more determination, resilience, honor, fortitude, hope, faith, joy, and love. In fact, if there was an event for "Passion for Life," they would all be awarded prestigious gold medals. I cherish each of my "breast friends."

Winning at breast cancer is not so much about our obstacles, but about our attitudes and how we overcome them. Being a survivor is all about enjoying life ... one day at a time.

Everyone is given lemons sometime in their life. Some are more bitter than others, but all are capable of being made into lemonade. It is turning them into something to enjoy that is most important—like pink lemonade.

Section III

Excerpts From CaringBridge

CaringBridge is a great tool that provides free websites to connect loved ones together from the onset of a critical illness through recovery. It is a nonprofit web service that is funded from tax-deductible donations. There are step-by-step instructions that are very easy to follow. They have twenty-four hour online support. You can choose from a wide variety of templates and even change the design with the seasons if you wish. There is also a place for you to post your favorite pictures of yourself, your family, and your experiences. More than twenty million families from around the world use CaringBridge each year.

I've included several of my journal entries and notes from friends to give you an idea of how CaringBridge works. My link is http://caringbridge.org/visit/marthalanier.

CHAPTER 9

Journal Entries

Writing my journal entries gave me an opportunity to share with my family and friends what I was experiencing.

SUNDAY, JUNE 01, 2008

I am more than ready to get this show on the road! Tomorrow (Monday) I begin the pre-op procedures and then Tuesday is the big day! You would think I was "nesting" the way I have been busy cleaning and getting things organized. I even dug up our winter flowers and replanted three beds in our front yard! Jim is loving this! I am well-prepared mentally, physically, and especially spiritually.

Mentally, I have not had any problems. In fact, since I was first diagnosed with cancer, I have had an opportunity to see my life from a much better view! Physically, I am now walking three miles in the neighborhood early every morning, and I'm drinking so much water to stay hydrated that I feel like I'm growing gills! Spiritually, my faith is stronger than ever. It has been strengthened by a wide variety of circumstances, especially throughout the past twelve months. I am doing my part, the surgeons will do theirs, and the rest is totally in God's hands.

In your prayers, please ask for the skills from my two surgical teams and for strength not just for me, but for Jim, my family, and friends. The Lord doesn't ever put on us more than we can handle. He obviously has a lot of confidence in me and I don't intend on letting Him down. Thank you for your prayers, support, and the great humor so many of you have shared. Your guestbook entries on CaringBridge and personal emails have meant the world to me. There is no doubt in my mind that I will have a speedy recovery and will soon be kicking my heels together. At my age, that is a feat in itself!

Martha

TUESDAY, JUNE 03, 2008

To All Our Friends and Family:

First off, we would like to thank you for all the thoughtful messages and prayers. Martha went into surgery at 8:00 this morning. Several lymph nodes were removed and the initial lab report indicates that they were benign. Obviously great news so far! Both doctors were very confident that the surgery was a complete success, but we will get the results from the pathology report sometime by the end of next week. Martha is doing as well as expected and is recovering comfortably thanks to a hefty dose of "happy drugs"!

The plastic surgeon will waste no time and have her up and walking tomorrow. We'll give more updates, so please keep checking in. Martha has also already read the many great e-mail messages you have sent through this site. Even if it's just a couple of words, they put a smile on her face.

Jim & Lauren

WEDNESDAY, JUNE 04, 2008

Today was a good day! Martha had her I.V. removed, walked three times on the third floor, and feels good. She even put makeup on ... you know Martha! She will probably come home Saturday. The doctors feel she is making wonderful progress. Thank all of you again for your prayers and support. We could not have done this without all of you. God does answer prayers and all usually ends well. We are blessed.

Jim

THURSDAY, JUNE 05, 2008

Well, today was even better than yesterday! Martha took a shower and washed her hair! Can you imagine how good that felt after three days in a hospital? We went for a good walk and she ate solid food, such as it is. She has had many visitors and calls.

Jim

FRIDAY, JUNE 06, 2008

Martha had a good day, but she was somewhat tired and spent the day resting. She was told that all the meds given to her during surgery were wearing off, so this is to be expected. She wanted me to tell everyone "hi" and thanks you for your prayers and good wishes. Her room looks like a florist shop.

She's coming home tomorrow (Saturday), so I will have my roomy, sweetheart, and soul mate back! God bless all of you for your concern, prayers, and love. Prayer does work!

Jim

SATURDAY, JUNE 07, 2008

Hooray! Martha is home! She is really washed out, but happy to be home and sleep in her own bed.

Jim

MONDAY, JUNE 09, 2008

This is a "red letter" day! Our prayers continue to be answered. Martha saw her surgeon today and received great news. Her final pathology report revealed negative results! There is no cancer in her lymph nodes and no other tumors were found! She had two more drainage tubes removed, leaving only one.

Jim

THURSDAY, JUNE 12, 2008

I am now one week and two days post-op and am cancer free! Each day I feel better and stronger. My energy level is gradually increasing and the discomfort is slowly decreasing. God continues to answer our prayers. I understand I was on quite a "high" for the first several days after surgery. Meds have a way of helping you feel better both mentally and physically. By Friday I started experiencing the effects of the surgery. Coming home on Saturday was a relief to Jim, yet somewhat scary for me. In the hospital I had a certain level of comfort and security.

Because I am such a control freak, after coming home, I felt the responsibility of keeping track of when I took pain meds and my antibiotic, as well as managing the care of my tubes. I was also aware of being active, yet not overdoing it. Only one tube remains, so in one week I have gone from feeling like an octopus with multiple tentacles to a stingray with just one. This last one will probably be removed later today or tomorrow.

One of the hardest things for me has been backing off and slowing down. As many of you know, this is not characteristic of my style. I usually stay in fast-forward. Before surgery one of my nurses told me that the first two weeks following surgery can determine the rate of my recovery. I am focusing on reading, resting, and writing in my daily journal. I look forward to my afternoon naps as "healing time" and consider this one of the perks of having surgery. I have two main limitations. For the first three weeks I can not raise my arms higher than my shoulders, which means not reaching for things on top shelves … which I never really wanted until I realized I now can't get to them. Also, for six weeks I cannot lift anything heavier than ten pounds. For someone who is so independent, I have learned to be creative.

Martha

SUNDAY, JUNE 15, 2008

My biggest accomplishment was getting the last tube removed last Friday. The nurse was fabulous! I never felt a thing! Yahoo!

I have had many more good days than bad and am amazed at how I have been able to move around, go up and down stairs, shower, and wash my hair. Except for occasional shooting pains here and there, the main discomfort has been a burning sensation caused from the nerves healing. This has decreased dramatically compared to this time last week, so I'm improving.

I have continued to journal, but realize my attention span is not very long. I will start working on a project or sit at my computer and in less than five minutes I either lose focus or energy. I am now realizing the importance of having patience and that the body requires more time to heal than I realized. At least I am getting in some good reading.

Martha

THURSDAY, JUNE 19, 2008

Two Weeks, Two Days Post-Op

Look out! I'm on the road again! Yesterday I was given the go-ahead to drive. Last night before dark, I headed out (alone) for a test drive in our neighborhood. Before I realized it, I was in downtown Cumming. I put down all of the windows, opened the sunroof, and turned the radio on full blast! Boy, did I feel free as a bird out of a cage! I even had the nerve to drive back home on (Highway) 400. Jim said I reminded him of a teenager with a new driver's license. I had a blast! Today I even drove by myself all the way down to my appointment by Northside Hospital.

Yesterday my plastic surgeon said he was extremely pleased with my recovery and progress. I only have a small amount of residual drainage, which he says is normal. The burning sensation continues to decrease a little more each day, but still remains throughout the night. He suggested that eliminating my afternoon nap would help. (At least I enjoyed them while I could.) In the morning I am now able to stand up fairly straight, but as the day progresses, my abdominal muscles and surgery sites tighten and I tend to bend forward. Every day I remind myself that I am so much better today than I was this time last week.

My breast surgeon gave me the fabulous news that the last remaining test results were negative and within normal ranges. He was amazed at how well I am feeling and getting around. He referred me to an oncologist for follow-up. Obviously I'm anxious to hear what she has to say, but I won't be seeing her for several weeks. There is no immediate rush since all of my reports were so good. Our prayers continue to be answered.

Martha

SUNDAY, JUNE 29, 2008

Three Weeks, Four Days Post-Op

Saturday, a week ago, I woke up feeling really good and decided I would drive the hour distance and attend the monthly meeting of the Georgia chapter of the National Speakers Association. Shortly after the meeting started, we passed the microphone to learn who was there and what they spoke on. This is the first time ever I have been given a standing ovation for just standing up and saying my name! Simply put, I was blown away by the reception I was given. The members are like my extended family. Just seeing everyone again was such a boost! There is simply no other medicine that can heal and speed a recovery faster than the love, warmth, and support of good friends and colleagues! Needless to say, I was totally drained by the afternoon, but it was well worth every ounce of energy I used to get me through the day. I will always savor and remember this experience and how everyone made me feel. Wow!

I had an appointment with my plastic surgeon on Wednesday. I always feel so much better when I see him. Just hearing him say that I am doing well and the incisions are healing nicely causes a sigh of relief that everything is okay. He said the burning sensations I am experiencing across my chest should keep decreasing and my energy increasing. Now that I am three weeks post-op, he started me on shoulder exercises. Although these aren't easy, I know they are important. Each day I am able to stretch higher.

On Friday I met my oncologist for the first time. My appointment lasted for over an hour as she went through every detail of my medical history and pathology reports. Based on the results, she said I was *not* a candidate for chemotherapy. I am basically cancer free at this time and the possible side effects of taking chemo could cause more harm than good. She started me on a relatively new drug called Femara. Its purpose is to reduce the risk of cancer returning to another part of my body. It is specifically for postmenopausal women who have been treated for early-stage breast cancer.

God has blessed me in so many ways. My goal is to pass these blessings on to others by speaking to as many groups as possible about facing challenges, taking control, and maintaining a positive attitude.

Martha

TUESDAY, JULY 15, 2008

Six Weeks Post-Op

I can't believe my surgery was six weeks ago today! On my walk this morning I thought about all that has happened since my surgery on June 3. I'm gradually increasing my distance and finished two miles today. Physically I am feeling really good, with only random aches and pains. The burning sensation I had been experiencing has finally gone away. What a relief! My abdomen is still partially numb and extremely tight, especially by the end of the day. I'm not complaining; it could be worse.

My plastic surgeon said now that I have reached the six-week mark, I no longer have any limitations. I can lift, reach, exercise, bike, and even swim. I'm proud to share that I have full mobility in both of my shoulders! I have truly been blessed with a smooth recovery. I feel my memory is getting sharper. I have been told to be patient because this is quite normal and to be expected after having the extent of surgery I had, plus what I have had to mentally process for the past three months.

During my experience with cancer, I have had an opportunity to meet some of the most incredible women who are also cancer survivors. There is an organization called The Wellness Community that offers a variety of free programs to cancer patients. So far I have gone to my first nutrition class where I learned how sugar affects cancer and the importance of eating fruits and vegetables. For someone who is allergic to the kitchen and who doesn't enjoy cooking, I'm learning new ways to prepare food. I even bought a vegetable steamer! Don't laugh! This is a new experience for me. Now I just have to find how to make some good sauces to make my veggies taste better. By the way, I welcome any recipes you might want to share. The Wellness Community offers two nutrition classes every month plus a wide variety of other interesting programs and exercise classes. I went to my first ever T'ai chi class and learned how to "meditate from my core" (which I first had to find). Tomorrow I will start the yoga classes. Man, am I going to be fit!

Last week Liz drove down from Spartanburg with our three grandsons to visit for several days. I had not seen her since Mother's Day, so her hugs and kisses were extra special. It was so much fun seeing the boys again. One night we all went out for dinner. We had Liz and her three boys, our other daughter, Lauren, her husband, and their two little girls, our son, Jim, and his wife and two little boys. The only one missing was Liz's husband. Yes, there were seven adults with seven grandchildren ranging in age from nine months to nine years! It meant so much having my family together!

Martha

WEDNESDAY, JULY 23, 2008

Seven Weeks Post-Op

What a difference each week makes! I can honestly say that at week seven, I am about 99 percent free from any discomfort, am feeling fabulous, and there isn't much I can't do. I have thoroughly enjoyed attending yoga classes, which is a new experience for me. I have now been to two classes and the stretching has helped tremendously. I especially look forward to the last fifteen minutes when we relax and meditate. I quickly learned after the first class not to lie flat on my back during this segment. At the end of my first class, the last thing I remember was lying on my mat, relaxing, listening to soft music, and taking slow deep breaths, when all of a sudden I heard a loud weird noise. I woke myself up snoring! The next class I made sure to lie on my side.

Because I've had such a fast recovery, my surgeon agreed that I will be strong enough to walk thirty miles in the Atlanta 2-Day Walk for Breast Cancer on September 20 and 21. Each walker is committed to collecting $1,000 in donations. Funds collected from this event are used locally. They not only provide education and research for breast cancer, but they also fund the programs, seminars, and exercise classes I enjoy attending. I have made the commitment to walk for It's the Journey, the non-profit organization sponsoring the Atlanta 2-Day Walk.

Regardless of what you may have recently heard in the news, self-exams (in addition to mammograms and ultrasounds) *are* a vital source for finding breast cancer. Early detection is the key that dramatically increases the chances for survival.

Martha

WEDNESDAY, JULY 30, 2008
Eight Weeks Post-Op

I'm so excited to share my latest news! I am now registered for the Atlanta 2-Day Walk, which is sponsored by the non-profit organization It's The Journey. On Saturday I went on my first training walk with some of the other walkers. All last week I had psyched myself up to be able to finish the six-mile route. Up until now, the most I had ever walked at one time was three miles in my neighborhood, so this was going to be a big challenge for me.

When I arrived at the site that morning, it was slightly overcast (which was great for walking) and I felt absolutely fabulous! I breezed past the three-mile mark and then past the six-mile mark. Would you believe I completed the entire twelve-mile course? Wow! I was sooooo excited! What was even more of a surprise was the fact that I didn't fall flat on my face the next day when I got out of bed. Actually, I felt pretty good! I am now confident that by September I'll be capable of completing the walk, and I'm equally excited knowing that the donations will help so many women.

Have I mentioned that my memory has finally returned? Well, let's just say that it is at least back to where it was *prior* to my surgery. I wish someone had told me weeks ago that deep breathing and rapid exhaling speeds the process of removing the lingering anesthesia out of your lungs.

My journey over the past several months has been an incredible experience. I now realize that eating healthy and exercising regularly make all the difference in the world about how I feel. I can actually say that I'm thankful for my wakeup call and having a second chance to enjoy life.

Martha

WEDNESDAY, SEPTEMBER 03, 2008

Three Months Post-Op

Never in my wildest dreams did I ever imagine that I would spend the entire summer of 2008 recovering from a mastectomy and reconstructive surgery. The results of my journey have truly been a miracle and I know prayers continue to be answered. Last night I read all of my guestbook and journal entries on CaringBridge. Then I read each of the cards and letters I had received. It brought back memories of the love and support I have received since I was first diagnosed with breast cancer.

It was five months ago that I first found the lump and it's been three months since my surgery. I realize now more than ever how lucky I am that my cancer was diagnosed early and that I didn't have to have chemo. Although I still have random pinches from nerves that continue to heal, I have had a remarkable recovery.

During the past two weeks I had follow-up appointments with each of my surgeons. My plastic surgeon scheduled the second phase of my reconstruction surgery for November 12. Small implants will be placed behind the TRAM tissue and my pec muscles. This will be done as an outpatient and will involve a short recovery time. I am so ready to get all of this behind me and move on. Although my breast surgeon was pleased with my progress, he gave me a lecture about having more patience about giving myself time to complete the healing process.

Several weeks ago I flew to New York to attend the annual convention of the National Speakers Association. Attendees had been asked to dress like a rock star during the opening event to kick off the theme,

"NSA Rocks!" I still can't believe I actually had the nerve to dress like Madonna! From the black lace ankle socks and heels up to my blonde wig, I could have passed for her double. I'll leave the rest for your imagination! I would have blended better with the crowd if I had not been one of only about fifty in costume out of the other 1,900 attendees!

It feels great being back to work and speaking again. I realize how much I honestly love what I do. I have added a new program where I share some of my experiences as a new breast cancer survivor. My goal is to help raise awareness by speaking to as many organizations as possible and help remove some of the fear associated with breast cancer.

Martha

TUESDAY, SEPTEMBER 30, 2008
Three and a Half Months Post-Op

I never would have believed I would walk thirty miles in a day and a half, but guess what? *I did it!* Walking in the Atlanta 2-Day Walk for Breast Cancer was the most incredible experience! There were over 1,200 participants and more than $1.1 million was raised for breast cancer research and support for survivors!

Thanks to many of you, my daughters and I raised just under $4,000 in just over two months! I designed t-shirts for us to wear, listing the names of the people we were walking for on the front, and the names of everyone who gave us donations making it possible for us to walk on the back.

For me, it was extra special to have Liz and Lauren walk with me, especially since this was my first year as a new survivor. We made it through the weekend with only several blisters and no major injuries other than the huge bruise I got on my left hip. Like usual, I was so busy talking, I never saw the three-foot tall concrete planter in the middle of the sidewalk. I had so much momentum, I think I may have actually moved it! I'll be wearing this colorful reminder for at least another week or two! At least I have a good story to add to my program about the importance of maintaining focus. It was both an honor and a thrill when

I was asked to speak during the closing ceremony. I shared my experience as a newcomer to breast cancer and how I have benefited from the programs sponsored by the funds raised from the walk. It is a weekend I will always remember!

Martha

MONDAY, NOVEMBER 03, 2008
Five Months Post-Op

October was an exciting month! Last week I was interviewed by CBS 46 News. The storyline was about breast cancer survivors who had been diagnosed with cancer after having a negative mammogram.

With Thanksgiving only weeks away, I realize how much I have to be thankful for this year. My cancer was caught early, my treatment was successful, I am cancer-free, I have so many new "breast friends," I have the most supportive family and friends, and I now have my priorities in order. Thanks to each of you for your support and encouragement. I wish you a warm and wonderful Thanksgiving.

Martha

WEDNESDAY, NOVEMBER 12, 2008

Martha had her second phase of reconstructive surgery today. She came through the procedure great and her surgeon was extremely pleased with the outcome. She is still groggy from the anesthesia, but is home and resting comfortably.

Jim

SUNDAY, NOVEMBER 30, 2008
Six Weeks Post-Op—Mastectomy and TRAM
Two Weeks Post-Op—Second Surgery

Since our previous journal entry, my last tube was removed, I had my two-week post-op checkup, and I continue to feel better every day. Initially, I underestimated this last procedure and quickly realized no surgery should be taken lightly. The hardest part for me again has been having patience during the healing process. For the past two weeks Jim has waited on me 24/7 and now has me totally spoiled. Even for such an independent person, I have thoroughly enjoyed being pampered.

Whoever said "silence is golden" obviously didn't have grandchildren! All seven of ours (ages one to nine-and-a-half) left this afternoon. We would much rather have them here, laughing and running through the house, than to have to deal with the silence. With five little boys and two little girls, there was never a dull moment! It was so much fun seeing all of those little cousins having so much fun together. Our three children, their spouses, one mother-in-law, and seven grandchildren were with us during Thanksgiving. All of the women totally took over my kitchen and prepared an absolutely fabulous Thanksgiving feast!

I can't believe it's already time to get out Christmas decorations and put up our tree. In just three weeks the silence will once again be replaced with giggles and excitement when most of our grandchildren will be here to celebrate Christmas!

Martha

FRIDAY, FEBRUARY 06, 2009
Eight Months Post-Op—Mastectomy and TRAM

It is already February and I feel like spring is just around the corner! I just realized it has been two months since I have posted an update. First of all, I am feeling fabulous! I saw my surgeon several weeks ago for follow-up from my surgery in November. He said I have no limitations and can do whatever I want. This was all Lauren and Liz (my daughters) needed to hear. They reissued their challenge for me to compete with them in the Aflac Iron Girl Sprint Triathlon. We were scheduled to do this last year, but obviously had to postpone it when I had my mastectomy. We have started training again and will compete on June 28 at Lake Lanier Islands. They have competed in triathlons before, but this will be my first. Please continue with your prayers as I get this bod in shape so I can keep up with them.

I am putting the finishing touches on the manuscript for my book, which should be available by late spring or early summer. It includes positive, informative, and humorous tips on having breast cancer. My goal is to encourage early detection and remove some of the fear many women associate with breast cancer.

Martha

WEDNESDAY, APRIL 1, 2009

Ten Months Post-Op—Mastectomy and TRAM

April 1, 2008, exactly one year ago, is the day I first discovered the lump. Little did I know it would be breast cancer. I realize there are so many things I have to be thankful for, such as finding it early while it was still small, going to a doctor who followed her intuition to have it tested, using two of the best surgical teams anyone could ever dream of having, and meeting some of the strongest and most remarkable women.

Within the past several weeks I have seen my internist, breast surgeon, new gynecologist, plastic surgeon, and oncologist. I am thrilled that after extensive exams, sticks, pokes, and prods, they all five agree I am in excellent physical condition.

They were especially supportive and excited when I told them I had registered for a First Timers Triathlon on June 6 and the Aflac Iron Girl on June 28. In fact, several said they may come to Lake Lanier Islands and cheer me across the finish line.

I know this is a tremendous undertaking, but I'm not one to turn down a challenge. My daughters are really putting me to the test this time. Up until about a week ago I was training on my treadmill and a stationary bike. Not to worry—I have now stepped up my training. Last week I joined Hearthstone Lodge Pool and Fitness Center, which is only about a ten-minute drive from home. Membership is only for the fifty-plus age group. Most are in their eighties and can kick my butt in the pool. One introduced herself as "eighty-one and still having fun." I love that they are all so friendly and have welcomed me into their group.

It has been a long, long time since I have been in a pool, much less swum laps. My immediate goal is to build my stamina and increase swimming the number of lengths before having to hang on the side to catch my breath. I obviously have my work cut out for me.

This past Saturday I bought my bike, helmet, and bike rack. I'm so excited, but oh so nervous about this part of the event. I had a hand-me-down bike growing up, but that was fifty years ago! The only other time I have ridden since then was about five years ago. We rented bikes during a vacation with our children and grandchildren. On my first ride, I forgot the brakes were on the handlebars and just tried pushing backwards on the pedals. (If you don't know what I'm talking about, ask your parents.) I ran straight into the curb, flipped over the handlebars and took about five layers of skin off of my left knee. My grandson had the nerve to say, "Why didn't you just use the brake if you wanted to stop?"

I was seriously thinking about buying knee and elbow pads to go with my helmet, but my daughter wouldn't let me. That didn't surprise me because she also said "no" to a bell, basket, streamers, and flag.

I'll keep you posted on my progress! By the way, please don't stop with the prayers. I can definitely use all of the help I can get.

Martha

Tuesday, June 9, 2009
One year, one week post-op

It's hard to believe it's been one year since my mastectomy. On Wednesday, June 3rd, we celebrated while vacationing at the beach in Florida with our son Jim, his wife Becky and the boys, Christopher and Michael. Jim gave me roses, took us all out to dinner and then we ate a delicious ice cream cake.

I celebrated again 3 days later by competing in my first sprint triathlon. It consisted of a 1/4 mile swim in Lake Lanier, biking 12 miles and running (I only walked) 3 miles. I was excited just to finish, but doubly excited because I finished in less than 2 hours. My official time was 1:59:50. Not bad for a 61 year old breast cancer survivor! Click on the

Photos link in the top banner for a picture of me crossing the finish line. (The clock is not the official time because it does not reflect the actual time recorded by the timing chip I wore on my ankle.)

I thought I did really great until I met Marge. She was 76 and this was also her first triathlon. Because we were in the same heat (the old timers), I knew I beat her in the swim. Then as I was leaving on my bike, she literally blew past me. I forgot about her until I saw her running up hill on her way to the finish line just as I was starting the run (walk). She was incredible!

Marge is my new hero and inspiration as I continue my training in preparation for the upcoming Aflac Iron Girl Sprint Triathlon. It is in less than 2 weeks on June 28th. I'm so excited that Liz and Lauren will be competing with me. This swim will be 1/3 mile, the bike is 18 miles and the run the same 3 miles. If anyone would have told me I would be doing this, I would have thought they were crazy. I have to admit I am having a blast and feel better than I ever have in my entire life.

I had hoped my book would have been released by now, but editing took longer than I anticipated. We are now anticipating it will be in late June. This has been an exciting year with the triathlons and my book being published. I'll let you know when *Pink Lemonade: Mastectomy Tips and Insights from a Breast Cancer Survivor* is released.

Thanks for your continued support and prayers. On my next update, I'll let you know how I did in the Iron Girl.

Martha

Monday, June 30, 2009

One year, one month post-op

On Sunday I finished my first official triathlon - the Aflac Iron Girl! The First Timers Tri I did several weeks ago was not a sanctioned triathlon and all events were shorter distances. The Iron Girl consisted of a 1/3 mile swim, 18 mile bike and 5K run/walk. I'm the first to admit it was a tough course and the 95 degree heat didn't help. The highlight for me was when I turned the corner and headed for the finish line, Liz and Lauren joined me and ran the last 100 yards with me. What a thrill!

The three of us were also selected by Iron Girl to be three of seven special interest participants and included with six pros who were also competing to be featured in a special, NBC Sports will air on Sunday, August 2nd from 2-3. We were interviewed individually on Saturday and then had cameras following us throughout each of the events on Sunday. Can I say pressure! There's nothing like a kick to your run when a motorcycle with a TV camera pulls up and joins you while you're sweating profusely and gasping for air while you're acting like there's nothing to it.

We had a blast. Our entire family was there to cheer us on including Jim, my son, Jim and his wife, Lauren's and Liz's husbands and all seven of our grandchildren. It is a day I will never forget.

I have to admit I now have "tri fever". My next competition is August 9th in the Acworth Tri. To top it off, yesterday Lauren upgraded to a newer bike and I bought her old one (I quickly realized my hybrid just isn't fast enough). This afternoon my daughter-in-law, Becky, called to say she registered for the Acworth Tri which will be her first. Then Lauren called tonight and said her husband bought a tri bike today and they are both registered to compete in the Greenville Tri in August with Liz and her husband. Jim and I will have babysitting duty for their total of 5 children.

I am feeling fabulous. Tomorrow I have a follow-up appointment with my surgeon and am confident he will give me a great report.

Watch out – tri fever is highly contagious. Two friends joined me in competing in the First Timers and one in the Iron Girl. Another friend in my mastermind group said she may want to compete next year. How about you?

Martha

APPENDIX
Checklist

When I was preparing for my surgery, I created this list and then made several copies. I put one in my purse for shopping and put another with my suitcase to use when I packed for the hospital.

What to do prior to surgery:

_____   Set up CaringBridge website

_____   Determine point of contact

_____   Create phone lists

_____   Collect mailing addresses

_____   Move items you use often that are currently on higher shelves down to waist-high level

_____   Make a collage of pictures of your family and friends

What to buy prior to surgery:

_____   Sudoku and crossword books (buy these soon and begin using now when going to your appointments)

_____   Thank you notes

_____   Stamps

_____   Journal

_____   Backrest pillow form / wedge pillow

_____   Tablet

_____   Nightshirt that buttons up the front

_____ Camisoles

_____ Button-up blouses

_____ Pants with elastic or drawstring waists

_____ Toupee tape

_____ Three boxes of candy for your nurses

What to take to the hospital:

_____ Wrap-around robe

_____ Slippers

_____ Makeup

_____ Hair dryer

_____ Toiletries

_____ Cell phone and charger

_____ Tablet

_____ Favorite framed pictures

_____ Printed jokes for nurses and visitors

_____ Three boxes of candy for three shifts of nurses

_____ _____

_____ _____

_____ _____

_____ _____

What You Can Do For Yourself

- **Don't panic**—Do your homework and learn as much as you can.
- **Don't be afraid to ask questions**—This is not the time to be hesitant or shy. Ask all of the questions you can think to ask. I promise there isn't one that is insignificant.
- **Go with your gut feeling**—We have a unique intuition system; now is a great time to use it.
- **Do your research**—Don't depend solely on your doctors. They will use their expertise to guide you, but it is your responsibility to be involved with the final decisions from diagnosis through recovery.
- **Write down your thoughts**—Often important thoughts are lost and forgotten just because no one ever bothered to put them in writing. Don't take a chance on trusting your memory.
- **Speak out loud**—Share your thoughts with a close friend who will listen and not give an opinion. Also, just by hearing ourselves say something, we create clarity.
- **Don't allow others to influence your decisions**—Give yourself permission to do what *you* want to do and not what you believe others think you should do.
- **Stay positive**—Avoid negative people. If people appear sad and depressed when they are around you, speak up and tell them you need their help in maintaining a positive attitude.
- **Stay busy and plan fun activities**—Work on your dream lists and everything else you can think of that you would like to do but haven't taken the time or money to do.
- **Eat healthy and nutritious foods**—You don't have to change everything, just become aware of what you are eating and make an effort to focus on eating healthy foods. One of the hardest things for me to do was give up sugar.

- **Get in the habit of exercising**—This is one of the best things you can do for yourself, both before and after surgery. Walking and moving around while you are in the hospital will increase the flow of blood and oxygen to your surgery sites and help with healing. Continue exercising after you get home. It will help your stamina, flexibility, heart and overall health.

- **Don't hesitate to ask for help even when you don't think you need it**—There are people who will jump at the chance to help you. Let them.

- **Be aware of the emotions your family and friends are experiencing**—Cancer affects them, too, just in a different way.

- **Use your resources**—This may come in the form of other breast cancer survivors. You will not find anyone else who is more understanding and supportive.

- **Write a list of questions you want to ask your doctors**—It is so easy to forget the questions once you are in the office or exam room. I often wrote them on my calendar on the day of my appointment on my BlackBerry. This way I could add new questions as I thought of them even days ahead of time. I knew I would always have my phone with me.

- **Make every day special**—Even if it is having personal time, going to yoga, having a manicure or pedicure, reading a good book, having lunch with a friend, taking a walk outside—whatever it is, make every day special.

What Family And Friends Can Do For You

You may want to share this book with your family and friends and let them read this segment. It is an easy way to show them how to help you.

- **Be positive**—Let her know you are going to be there for her.
- **Be prepared**—With one out of eight women being diagnosed with breast cancer in their lifetime, *now* is the time for you to prepare yourself for a response when a friend or family member tells you they have been diagnosed with breast cancer. Rather than showing shock, surprise, or pity, be prepared to be strong for her.
- **Be present and in the moment**—Give her your full attention and look her in the eye. Don't go into lengthy conversations and tell her about a friend with a similar experience. Right now it is all about her.
- **Listen more than speak**— If she is willing talk, be attentive and listen. If she doesn't want to talk, don't push.
- **Be supportive**—Regardless of how badly you want to offer your opinion, every woman approaches breast cancer differently. This is *her* life and *her* choices. It is always easy to think about what we would do in a specific situation but we really don't know until it actually happens to us. It may be helpful to offer suggestions she may not have thought about but let her decisions be hers.
- **Confirm what you are hearing**—Repeat important phrases she has said to make sure you understand what she means.
- **Be *specific* when offering to help**—Don't just ask, "What can I do?" Be specific in what you offer to do. You may say, "I'm going to bring dinner over your first night home from the hospital." She'll let you know if this offer has already been made.

Suggestions:

- Coordinate meals with neighbors and friends for after she gets home from the hospital.
- Go with her to doctors' appointments for company and as a second pair of ears.
- Go to the grocery store on a specific day.
- Drive her to appointments.
- Take her to lunch, for a leisurely drive, to a movie, on a short shopping trip, or help her run her errands.
- Offer to come and visit (Note: Listen more than talk and don't outstay your welcome—even a short visit in the beginning can be exhausting for her. She will never speak up and tell you to leave because she doesn't want to appear rude).
- Bring lunch for the two of you.
- Help with household chores such as cleaning or unloading the dishwasher or better yet, give a gift of a one-time house-cleaning service (I wasn't able to push a vacuum cleaner for several months).
- Help with children—Drive carpools, baby-sit, entertain them or give children quiet toys or games.
- Help with a pet—Walk her dog at specific time or board or be responsible for the pet's care for while she is in the hospital.
- Provide her with humor—Bring her joke books or comedy movies; email her jokes and funny YouTube links. Remember that laughter is the best medicine.
- Send frequent upbeat emails—Something as simple as, "thinking of you" lets her know you care. You may want to send her a cheery e-card.
- Bring flowers—If they are fresh-cut, make sure they are already in a vase.

- Take her a goody bag of snacks on the day of her surgery—
  My "breast friend" Debbie did this for me so my visitors
  could enjoy a snack when they stopped by to visit. My husband, children, grandchildren and friends loved this. I admit
  I ate my share as well.
- Offer encouragement—Give her kind and cheerful words
  frequently to show your support and encouragement.
- Don't ask her how she is feeling. This directs her to respond
  with comments on her pain, discomfort, or emotions. Just
  ask, "How are you?" She can respond to this by saying anything from being ready to get out of the house, go shopping,
  take a nap, sit and visit, or hundreds of other things. This is
  more general and can relate to almost anything, including
  her feelings, if that is what she wants to talk about.
- Treat her the same as you always have—Having breast cancer or a mastectomy doesn't change *who* she is.

Links and References

American Cancer Society
http://www.cancer.org

National Cancer Institute
http://www.cancer.gov/cancertopics/types/breast

Insurance coverage for reconstructive surgery
(Government information)
http://www.dol.gov/dol/topic/health-plans/womens.htm

American Institute for Cancer Research
(great for general information including recipes)
http://www.aicr.org

Nutrition and other facts
(informative website)
http://www.caring4cancer.com

Caring Bridge
http://www.CaringBridge.org

Atlanta Two-Day Walk for Breast Cancer
http://www.ItsTheJourney.org

Susan G. Komen for the Cure
http://ww5.komen.org

The Wellness Community National Headquarters
http://www.TheWellnessCommunity.org

Turning Point Women's Healthcare, Alpharetta, GA
http://www.MyTurningPoint.org

American Family Life Assurance Company of Columbus
http://www.Aflac.com

About The Author

Martha is an accomplished and sought-after speaker who has entertained and inspired audiences nationwide to live better, more fulfilling lives by overcoming the obstacles and fears they face. Ironically, in April 2008, she faced her own seemingly enormous obstacle when she found a lump in her right breast. Diagnosed with *stage 1 infiltrating ductal carcinoma,* Martha began a frightening, somewhat painful, at times humorous, and eventually enlightening experience as she dealt with everything that having breast cancer entails.

This mother of three and grandmother of seven has an incredible zest for life. With her enviable gift for finding joy in every day she lives, and her insatiable appetite for learning, she sought information about every aspect of living with breast cancer. Using both her newfound knowledge and passion for sharing, Martha wrote *Pink Lemonade: Mastectomy Tips and Insights from a Breast Cancer Survivor.*

Martha lives in North Georgia with her husband, Jim, whom she met in fifth grade. When not on the speaking circuit, she enjoys playing with her grandchildren and staying healthy by training for and competing in sprint triathlons (in the 60-64 age group).

Acknowledgments

Once total strangers, the many breast cancer survivors I have met through my journey have immediately become close friends as if we had known each other all of our lives. We are linked with a bond no woman ever wants to have, but once connected, we appreciate the love, compassion, comfort, and support that is included with this lifetime membership.

It amazes me that when you need help, friends just seem to automatically appear. Whether you brought dinner, sent me jokes and You-Tube videos, took me to lunch, visited me in the hospital or at home, sent cards, called, offered encouragement or supported me in writing this book —I love you all. I would like to thank you individually but you know who you are and what you mean to me.

Everyone I came in contact with at Northside Hospital Atlanta—the lab, x-ray department, admissions, surgical staff, nurses and techs—treated me with kindness and respect. My nurses on the 3rd floor were not only thoughtful and considerate but provided exceptional care and treated me royally.

My yoga instructor, Melba Black introduced me to a world of stretches, breathing techniques and quiet meditation. With her expertise, I was able to gently stretch my tight abdominal muscles and extend my arms high above my head after my surgery.

Robin Benardot, FD, LD who taught me which foods to avoid and which foods I need to eat every day. She helped change my poor eating habits of sweets and fast food to well-balanced meals. Because I don't enjoy cooking, she taught me easy-to-follow recipes and how to juice my fruits and veggies with a Vita-Mix.

Most of all I am forever grateful for my doctors: Dr. Colleen Austin, Dr. J. Patrick Luke, Dr. Phillip Beegle and Dr. Valerie Wender. I treated my cancer knowing that I had selected the most experienced, brilliant and extraordinary medical teams. Because of the expertise in each of their specialized fields, I was confident I would receive the best care possible.

Contact and Order Information

Every week Martha is contacted by women who have questions or who just want to talk. Because so many survivors were generous in talking with her when she was newly diagnosed, she wants to return the favor. Please feel free to contact her by phone or email. She would also enjoy hearing from you if you have comments about the book or your own experiences.

Contact Information:
Martha Lanier
4990 Magnolia Creek Drive
Cumming, GA 30028

770-886-6033

Martha@MarthaLanier.com
http://www.Martha Lanier.com

Pink Lemonade – Mastectomy Tips and Insights from a Breast Cancer Survivor is available in the following formats:
Paperback $15.95 (plus shipping and handling)
Downloadable eBook $9.95

Order Now
By Phone: 770-886-6033
By Email: order@PinkLemonadeBook.com
Buy Online: http://www.PinkLemonadeBook.com
By Mail: Martha Lanier
        4990 Magnolia Creek Drive
        Cumming, GA 30028
Bulk Orders Available

CPSIA information can be obtained at www.ICGtesting.com
Printed in the USA
LVOW041054020113

313994LV00001B/3/P

9 780981 975801